FOOD REBELS, GUERRILLA GARDENERS, AND SMART-COOKIN' MAMAS

FOOD REBELS, GUERRILLA GARDENERS, AND SMART-COOKIN' MAMAS

FIGHTING BACK
IN AN AGE OF INDUSTRIAL AGRICULTURE

MARK WINNE

BEACON PRESS
BOSTON

Beacon Press
Boston, Massachusetts 02108-2892
www.beacon.org

Beacon Press books
are published under the auspices of
the Unitarian Universalist Association of Congregations.

19 18 17 16   8 7 6 5 4 3

This book is printed on acid-free paper that meets the uncoated paper ANSI/NISO
specifications for permanence as revised in 1992.

Text design and composition by Wilsted & Taylor Publishing Services

Library of Congress Cataloging-in-Publication Data
Winne, Mark.
  Food rebels, guerrilla gardeners, and smart-cookin' mamas: fighting back in an
age of industrial agriculture / Mark Winne.
     p. cm.
  Includes bibliographical references.
  ISBN 978-0-8070-4737-8 (paperback : alk. paper)
  1. Food supply. 2. Nutrition policy. 3. Agriculture and state. I. Title.
  HD9000.5.W485 2010
  363.8—dc22   2010013436

*This book is dedicated to
all the smart-cookin' mamas of Austin,
the guerrilla gardeners of Cleveland,
the hard-working farmers of Connecticut,
and every food rebel in North America
who ever refused to accept fate.
You are, as Richard Wright once said, on
"the side that feels life most,
the side with the most humanity."
Don't ever stop fighting back.*

CONTENTS

PART I

AUTHORITY OR FREEDOM?

Today, people are persuaded more than ever that they have perfect freedom, yet they have brought their freedom to us and laid it humbly at our feet. . . . And we alone shall feed them. . . . Oh, never, never can they feed themselves without us! No science will give them bread so long as they remain free. In the end they will lay their freedom at our feet, and say to us, "Make us your slaves, but feed us."

—FYODOR DOSTOEVSKY, *The Brothers Karamazov*

As a food activist for nearly forty years, I have had days when I feel like I'm riding the perfect wave. Farmers' markets are busting out all over, everybody I talk to seems to be gardening, and the media's desire for organic and local food stories appears insatiable. It's during those moments that I feel like I'm standing high and handsome on a shiny surfboard skating across an unfolding curl of warm ocean water. There's an exhilarating sense of building momentum as the wave pulls energy from boundless coastal pools to form an ever-ascending crest. The force beneath me is gentle but magnificent, purposeful but wild with enthusiasm.

Although my career has provided enough moments like these to believe that the future might be better than the past, more often than not I find myself paddling in an angry sea where the threat of failure is far greater than the thrill of success. Experience has taught me that the industrial food system has become a tsunami that might very well engulf everything in its path. Big food corporations, unsustainable farming operations, and all their minions cannot check their momentum, nor do they want to. They are propelled by the seismic shocks that created them and are preserved by the failure of others to resist them. The wave that carried me, a nimble surfer on his dream ride, can easily turn hostile, hurling me onto shore. There I can lie, broken and beaten, my board shattered into a hundred pieces, or I can rise up, lick my salty wounds, and begin again.

This is a tale of the struggle that awaits. This is a tale of the choices we can make. As Hamlet said, "The readiness is all."

CHAPTER 1
A FOOD STORY FOR OUR TIMES
November 2020

I didn't care anymore. It wasn't only the morning fog slowly lifting from my head that had robbed me of the desire to fight. It was more than that. A heavy blanket of lethargy had suffocated the passion that once fueled me. To continue the struggle was insane. To surrender was all that remained.

Like a poultice for the psyche, my coffee's silky warmth brought momentary hope that something might yet push back the gloom. It was strong enough to deliver the required jolt; the rich aroma tickled the edges of my grief, evoking images of canopied Guatemalan hillsides and tree-dappled light; the full-bodied taste was as the fair trade, worker-owned coffee label promised: "Incomparable flavor, justly compensated." But the push back against despondency barely lasted half a cup. I could not conceal the truth from myself—I had caved. I had bought the dark, roasted beans at Mega-Shop, not from the socially just company of only ten worker-owners. The nation's biggest retailer's promise was eerily similar to that of the fair trader. The coffee was sustainably produced, the compensation paid to the growers was above the country of origin's prevailing wage, and the taste—well, it was not likely that even an educated coffee-sipping palate could discern the difference. But the price! God help us. It was 30 percent less than that of the good guys' coffee.

Not even the caramel hue lent to the coffee by the cream, or the sweet lick of honey, lightened my mood. The dairy conglomerate, Milk Max, had won its decade-long battle with the U.S. Department of Agriculture to label its milk "organic." Its 1,000 or so factory farm members, milking a minimum of 5,000 cows each, kept their animals confined, away from grass, fed on a mash made from certified biological by-products. The USDA was forced to approve these methods in the face of political pressure stemming from the current national food emergency.

A network of dairy pipelines now snaked across the country from the western high plains to the nation's metropolitan areas, sites of the mega-processing plants. Since trucking costs had gone through the roof, the federal government had subsidized the multibillion-dollar network as an energy conservation measure. In compliance with the national food czar's directives, local and state governments exercised eminent domain to seize private property and even turn over public lands to private operators to construct the web of steel. Initially, local resistance to the pipelines had been stiff. Peaceful protests had soon become more agitated. Angry mobs had resorted to rock throwing and the occasional Molotov cocktail. Guerrilla-style gangs (reminiscent of tree-spikers, who many years ago had attempted to thwart logging operations) had inflicted millions of dollars of damage at pipeline construction sites. And at least one life had been lost, when a heavy equipment operator failed to spot a young woman who had thrown herself in front of a giant earthmover.

But the outbreaks had subsided as the public resigned itself to the hopelessness of the struggle. A feeble set of lawsuits brought by the few remaining public interest law groups had been swiftly dismissed by the courts. Scattered bands of saboteurs roaming the countryside had been quickly rounded up. They had been easily identified by round-the-clock surveillance of the remaining small dairy farms that, in violation of the national food czar's decree, continued to sell milk directly to their doggedly loyal customers. The saboteurs were the ones seen on monitoring cameras bicycling to these farms to fill their own hodgepodge assortment of glass containers with organic, unpasteurized milk.

I had tried to avoid Milk Max, the industrial milk behemoth, by switching to soy-based creamers and drinks. But after MongoPlant had completed its takeover of all soybean producers, forcing the remaining holdouts, with the backing of federal regulators, to use genetically modified seed, I had returned to the Milk Max product line, perceiving it to be the lesser of two evils.

The honey in my coffee, the last remnant of anything produced locally by a small business, was itself threatened. The honey producers in my region of northern New Mexico were succumbing to a loss of water rights and land to developers in the expanding urban zones. The coup de grace had come slowly, with the loss of the farming and ranching skills that had sustained these small communities for 400 years. Disdainful young people who had no time for the "old ways" were hemorrhaging from the villages to the cities. The aging but still feisty Hispanic farmers who came to what was now the shriveled remnant of a once-vibrant farmers' market had lost that twinkle in their eyes. Their talk was less about their quirky forms of resistance— giving a passing Anglo tourist the wrong directions when one accosted them by the roadside—and more about recently deceased compadres whose children were putting the land up for sale. I had felt the change coming. I had watched one locally produced agricultural product after another pass slowly into extinction. Now even honey, the most local and most unassuming of nature's gifts—given freely and with so little required of humans in return—would soon become nothing more than roadkill on the industrial food system's highway.

Hoping my mood would improve with a walk in the garden, I grabbed my hat and coat and set off on my regular morning inspection tour. A light frost had nipped the tops of the tomatoes, peppers, and eggplant. That was as I had expected, since the thermometer was hovering around freezing just before dawn. It wasn't nature's little jabs, which gardeners learn to roll with, that unnerved me; it was the discomfiting realization that this first frost had come nearly a month past the "normal" frost date.

Extending the growing season as a result of global warming hadn't seemed so bad at first—the tomatoes yielded longer; late-maturing melon varieties were easier to grow. But my bemusement soon yielded to concern and then to the chilling fear that the seasons would decompose into nothing more than spaces marked on a calendar. Although plant scientists had recently reported success with the first orange grove in southern Colorado, the milder seasons had also brought less rain and snow. The time and cost associated with managing the irrigation system had begun to sap my physical energy as well as my pocketbook. Plant diseases and insects I had never seen before were starting to appear. And like other parts of the food chain, many of the smaller seed suppliers were evaporating in the changing economic climate, as the major seed corporations bought them out at ten cents on the dollar. Many had simply closed up shop in the face of declining interest in fruit and vegetable gardening. In what I surmised was a futile attempt to stave off the inevitable, one formerly independent seed house had sold out to MongoPlant. It proceeded to introduce an entire line of bioengineered vegetable seeds that, according to the description in the catalog, appeared to be tolerant to virtually every ailment that had ever afflicted the planet's flora. Apparently the belief in engineering our way around climate change was catching on.

Getting down on my knees to extract weeds from the cabbage patch was now a chore rather than a delight. It wasn't the ache in my aging joints, but rather a kind of mocking self that had moved into my consciousness. "What's the point?" it laughed at me. "You know your efforts are fruitless, you silly old man. This stuff is being grown cheaper, faster, and even better elsewhere. Why sweat so much? Why lose sleep over the weeds, the water, or the pests? You know that all is taken care of now. You can get in your car, you fool, and drive to the Mega-Shop for everything you want. Or if you still think that the Big Food corporations have placed the planet at risk, you can take your righteous ass down to Whole Wonders. Take up golf, play bridge—but don't waste your time growing food."

I knew "he," that voice in my head, was right. Even though I was theoretically capable of serving him an eviction notice, I couldn't shake him loose. And just in case I had preserved even a modicum of hope that we would triumph over Big Food, or at least be allowed to pretend that we were self-sufficient, he delivered the unkindest blow of all: "Besides, you pathetic holdout," he said with a smirk, "who's going to tend this garden, or any garden, for that matter, when you're gone? Your children? They don't want any part of it. They see no point in such silly labor now that all their needs are met."

The visit to the garden had only deepened my depression. I collapsed in front of the television, as mindless entertainment was all that I could manage. But instead of finding relief with a *MASH* rerun, I tuned to CNN. To my surprise it was broadcasting a debate between the new secretary of agriculture, Dr. Alston Whitlaw, and the executive director of the Local Foods Preservation Society, Kendell Derry. The subject of the debate was the hotly contested 2020 national farm bill, now titled the Freedom from Want and Concern Act.

Directing her lovely blue eyes toward the camera, moderator Penny Fryer tossed her blond locks past her black eyeglass frames as she began her introduction. "Dr. Whitlaw is America's newly appointed secretary of agriculture and the first person in the nation's history to be assigned the position of food czar."

That so few people had objected to this second and more potent title had struck me as odd. In the past, drug czars and energy czars had come and gone, and the absolute power vested in them by the term *czar* had been laughingly dismissed by the general public. Not this time. The hopes of a frightened population to deliver it from what had been billed as a pending disaster were riding on the Harvard PhD's shoulders. Indeed, Whitlaw's stern image, his perfectly coiffed, professorial head of wavy gray hair, commanded both attention and respect. His abundant academic credentials included advanced degrees in agronomy, economics, and human nutrition.

Yet there was something in his eyes that suggested compassion, a trait most likely cultivated during his post-college years spent in a Catholic seminary. His smile in response to Fryer's opening was engaging, but the gaze that locked on the camera contained more than a hint of imperiousness. Overlooked in Fryer's recitation of Whitlaw's impressive résumé were his multiple corporate and philanthropic affiliations, including a seat on both the MongoPlant Corporation, the global seed monopoly, and the Pates Foundation, the nation's largest philanthropy, boards, numerous university trusteeships, and a stint at the World Bank.

Assuming the role of yin to Whitlaw's yang was Derry, a slightly built figure wearing granny glasses whose shaven head and gentle visage made him appear more monk-like than formidably intelligent. The camera's close-ups revealed stray threads and small abrasions in his tweedy jacket, which had become his constant and much-caricatured companion during his 10,000-mile media march back and forth across America.

If Fryer's introduction of Whitlaw had been unctuous, her delivery as she presented Derry was decidedly cool. "Kendell Derry has written ten books on the subject of food, agriculture, and," she paused, raising her eyebrows, "the human spirit." Accelerating into a rapid-fire mode, she condensed the remainder of Derry's biography into a few tight-lipped fragments, "National Academy of Science...numerous teaching fellowships...sustainable development specialist." But with a look normally reserved for the moment when you discover puppy puke on your new Gucci pumps, Fryer paused for a second before saying, "Mr. Derry is also an organic grower on his family's thirty-acre farm in central Ohio."

"Mr. Derry," Fryer began the questioning, "you have proposed an alternative to the administration's farm bill that would shift the United States into what you and your allies call 'sustainable forms' of food production and locally controlled food distribution systems—what some critics have labeled 'centrally planned local economies.' Nine billion humans are projected to inhabit the globe by 2050, and the numbers of farms and farmers have reached an all-time low. How do you propose to feed a hungry world with the kind of food system that has been on the decline since the early twentieth century?"

"Food production in America," responded Derry, "depends increasingly on nonsustainable inputs—for instance, petro-chemical fertilizers and excessive use of water in areas where it is in short supply. This system produces lots of food, yes, but it is depleting finite resources and poisoning the environment. Because more consumers are aware of these conditions, the demand for sustainably produced food is at an all-time high. People want good food, which is food that is healthy, green, fair, and affordable. Our current system of food production and distribution is not delivering that."

Fryer, whose brow had been deeply furrowed during the time that Derry spoke, turned with a relaxed if not seductive air to Whitlaw and asked, "How, Dr. Whitlaw, do you respond to these *interesting* ideas?"

"Thank you, Penny," said Whitlaw, graciously acknowledging the host at the same time as he leaned aggressively in Derry's direction. "First off, I want to say how much I admire Kendell's work and his lifelong passion for justice and sustainability. But I do believe that his ideas contain more than trace of naïveté, especially in the face of the crisis that is now gripping the planet. Food prices have risen nearly 15 percent per year in the U.S. and at two to three times that rate in developing nations. Food riots, food shortages, and shrinking agricultural land are, as any cognizant person knows, the order of the day. Science and technology have made enormous strides in allowing farmers across the world to grow more food on less acreage than ever before. In 1950 we needed one farmer for every 27 people in the U.S.; today we only need one farmer for every 144 people. And we are doing that on less land—7.9 acres of farmland per person in 1950 and only 3.1 acres today. We should be celebrating the advances in agricultural sciences and technology, not blocking them as Kendell and his allies are attempting to do. His farm bill might serve an elite group of his followers, but will push billions of others further into hunger."

Fryer swiveled her chair to face Derry. "Mr. Derry, until a few months ago I was a loyal shopper at the downtown farmers' market. Though it's no secret that I make a good salary, I found the prices exorbitant! The average American, let alone a lower-income American, can't pay $8 for a pound of tomatoes, whether they are organic or not. It's one thing to ask people to give up their country club memberships to eat good food, but these prices may mean I have to give up sending my children to college."

Derry had encountered hostility to his ideas before. This was nothing new. But the long days on the road carrying the flag for a localized and sustainable food system appeared to be taking their toll. Fryer's skeptical gaze and Whitlaw's condescending smile were bringing visible beads of perspiration to Derry's forehead. In virtually inaudible gasps, he tried to respond. "We have ceded control of our seed production to MongoPlant. . . . MacBurger's, in spite of its overrated salads and posted calorie counts, feeds us food that's killing us, but, because of its multibillion-dollar advertising campaign, is practically the only place Americans eat out anymore. . . . Mega-Shop is 'greenwashing' us with products that are grown on factory-size farms that are organic in name only. . . . And the decisions about our food—what we eat, what we pay, how it's grown—are made by a small oligarchy of political and food industry representatives, now led by, of all things, a 'czar.'"

Both Fryer and Whitlaw eyed Derry patronizingly. "Kendell," Whitlaw began, speaking with the patient voice of a parent appealing to a wayward toddler, "millions have been drawn to your cause, in spite of the fact that you offer little more than hard work and faith. Billions, however, are following me and trusting in my authority because I am using the miracle and mystery of science and technology to produce food in ways they may not understand, but are willing to accept because they feed them. Genetically modified organisms have yet to bring about the biological holocaust that your advocates have asserted will occur. Moreover, MongoPlant's new seed varieties have opened up marginal agricultural land to food production and enabled African farmers to earn a profit for the first time in decades.

"The MacBurger's chain that you berate is wildly successful—a $3.5 billion profit, up 12.7 percent from the year before—because it is cheap and gives people what they want. Over 27 million customers eat at MacBurger's each day; do you think there's something wrong with them? And since you're also concerned about social justice, you must know that MacBurger's has made millionaires out of more black and Hispanic franchise owners than any other business.

"Food safety problems are killing thousands of people every year and making millions more sick. The people want to be protected but there is no one to trust other than the regulators and now me, since the president's assignment of food czar also carries with it the title of chief regulator. Like the need for larger farms, larger equipment, more expensive technology, seed, and inputs, food safety will mean more consolidation in farming and other food industries. A capital-intensive food system will be required because the public's safety cannot be compromised."

"The people want a voice because we live in a democracy," sputtered Derry in an attempt to regain his footing. "They don't want mega-corporations dictating the terms of the food they eat. Consumers are human beings, not little consumption automatons. Given a reasonable choice and opportunity, they want food to come directly from nature, not through a system that is highly manipulated by technology and controlled by only a few corporations. They want freedom of choice and the opportunity to express that choice. Isn't that what makes us human?"

With his eyes riveted on the camera lens, Whitlaw had the posture of a man about to issue an edict. "Kendell Derry and his followers are trying to maintain a system that may serve the elite few, but will fail the masses. As you know, the nation's major antihunger organizations have already signed off on my proposal to further support the consolidation of the food industry and the adoption of capital-intensive, high-technology solutions. They know the people want first and most of all to be fed. If they are not, political instability will result. And we're not talking just about the poor here. I'm willing to predict that most consumers will subscribe to our plan and put aside their values willingly when they realize that it is easier to submit to the nation's food authorities. They will trade free choice for material comfort and gladly relinquish their treasured freedom for the certainty of food."

Derry was visibly stunned by this pronouncement, and even Fryer's perpetual glow had faded. The shock of what Whitlaw was suggesting had apparently sucked the oxygen from the studio, holding everyone in a state of suspension. The debate was drawing to a close, but Fryer looked as if she would not be capable of ending the broadcast with her perky signature closing, "Goodnight and hugs and kisses to all." She turned instead to Derry as if pleading for guidance.

At that moment Derry's defeated look gave way to a gentle smile. His stooped shoulders straightened sharply and he leapt to his feet with a joy that startled the formerly imperturbable Whitlaw. Though the "czar" had come to embody all that Derry found hollow and fallen in this world, he gave the large man a bear hug and kissed him on the cheek. Doing the same to the still-shocked Fryer, Derry jogged offstage. The credits rolled across the images of Fryer and Whitlaw sitting on the set in silence as the show's theme song played.

I sat in my chair, the beer can I'd opened at the beginning of the debate still nearly full. What had happened? Had Derry simply grown frustrated and, rather than surrender, decided to declare victory and go home? Had he genuinely earned more debating points and won the contest? But then it dawned on me: Derry hadn't so much won as realized that Whitlaw, like the enterprise he stood for, would be defeated by his own illusion of omnipotence. It wasn't a case of whether Whitlaw's system would triumph over Derry's or vice versa. The question came down to the ability of democracy and individual freedom to resist, even when the claim is made by truly credible forces that we must submit in order to survive. Both sides had thrown down the gauntlet, and with my sense of purpose renewed, I grabbed my gloves and sprinted for the garden.

CHAPTER 2

THE FIGHT FOR THE SOUL OF THE AMERICAN FOOD SYSTEM

The way we understand the struggle for control of our food system will determine the way we fight the battle. To that end we need an analysis that is balanced and relies as much on the evidence as it does on our values. We must, however, have a clear appreciation of what's at stake. Though we may rightfully say that food is an equal partner in the holy trinity that includes air and water, it is, after all, *just* food. It is hard to argue with the fact that there is enough of it, and that the real challenge in providing equitable access to affordable calories lies primarily in the realm of distribution. But at another level the fight might be more than that. It might be that, to paraphrase William Blake, the road to the palace of wisdom is paved with food. Equally important as what is on our plates is what it says about who we are and how we live our lives.

The global food wars of the last fifty years have wrought little intentional human damage. Nevertheless, hundreds of millions of people have died from hunger; malnourishment has diminished the lives of hundreds of millions more; an untold number of lives have been cut short by the ravages of unhealthy eating and/or over-eating; and food-borne illnesses and man-made chemicals have killed or sickened millions more. Ironically, food, that life-sustaining force, may have, by dint of being too little, too much, or too tainted, taken more lives than all the weapons of post–World War II humankind.

It's not surprising that with so much at stake, people are continually formulating and reformulating strategies to reduce—or hopefully, one day, end—food's capacity to truncate human life. At the same time, individual or small-group attempts to address these problems on a scale that might make a difference have been largely supplanted by institutional efforts. Whether in the form of big government, big industry, big foundations, or big academia, institutional forces are working feverishly to influence our food systems.

Accompanying the decline of the individual and the ascendancy of the institution has been the rise of suspicion of motive. The food corporation that makes record profits as food prices soar hardly earns the respect and admiration of those who advocate for affordable food for all. Conversely, the corporation that keeps its prices low at the expense of low wages, meager health benefits, and a compromised environment will not secure the praise of those who want fair labor practices and sustainably produced products. Researchers and agricultural corporations who develop and market genetically modified seed contend that their products will feed a "hungry world." At the same time those who believe genetically modified organisms are unsafe, untested, and unsound vigorously oppose their development and dissemination. Food safety regulators and advocates are under the gun to protect the public safety in the face of a continual onslaught of food product recalls, and human (and animal) illnesses and deaths. But attempts to stiffen regulations often drive up costs for many farmers, processors, and distributors who can't afford to comply with higher standards. Judgments abound, people take sides, and every side thinks it has the magic bullet that will cure the world's ills. "If only they'd listen to me" is the usual refrain.

As the parable in the first chapter suggests, the world of food is changing rapidly and will take on forms in the future that we cannot even imagine. Is the story of the end of a sustainable, localized, and more intimate food system improbably futuristic, simply the nightmarish visions of a feverish author? Is the face-off between good and evil nothing more than a Hollywoodesque dramatization that suppresses the innumerable shades of gray that always lie between the white hats and the black hats?

As the food wars heat up—as evidenced by, among other things, the avalanche of food books, films, and blogs—it does appear as if the battle lines have been drawn between two major camps. The first and by far the most formidable, in terms of numbers, resources, and sheer dominance, is what we loosely call the industrial food system. To put it simply, it is the system from which most of us eat whether we like it or not, or whether we know it or not. It is highly organized, rational, efficient, and possesses a singular focus on the financial bottom line as both organization and management values. Though the word *industrial* implies a kind of lockstep adherence to the mass production, capital- and energy-intensive models of all industrial systems—whether they're manufacturing cars, computers, or pretzels—this food system is not necessarily the heartless brute lacking in the softer human sensibilities that some think. While it may be difficult at times to separate truth from fiction in a typical food industry press release, these corporate behemoths are, after all, comprised of nothing more than average people who feel, breathe, and think like other average people.

A recently retired CEO of my acquaintance, a man who ran one of the nation's largest food service corporations, has been devoting his time, expertise, and personal resources to the development of a regional food system including local farmers' markets and the development of food stores in underserved communities. Yes, he's also learning how to play the guitar and attending Zen retreats—such are the options of the privileged—but his retirement pursuits are sincere, effective, and not a late attempt to get right with his God. In fact, during the latter portion of his business career, he pushed his company hard to buy as much locally and sustainably produced food as possible. In the end, he had as much heart and soul as anybody else. I just had to scratch beneath the surface (and my stereotypes) to find it.

THE ALTERNATIVE FOOD SYSTEM

The other food camp is the alternative food system. While no easier to stereotype than the industrial food system, it is "alternative" because it has indeed evolved as a distinctively different model of food production, processing, and distribution, and in comparison to the industrial system, is a minority player, perhaps still an upstart. For some, the "alternativeness" expresses itself in direct opposition to the industrial food system, while others see it merely as a means to promote a more value-based approach to food, farming, and community.

What are its tenets? In general, the alternative food system produces food that does not harm the environment or human beings. But more than "doing no harm," alternative means managing the food system in a sustainable fashion—not depleting the natural resources upon which our food system depends, thus rendering those resources unusable by future generations. The alternative system also accounts for energy use, especially of nonrenewable sources such as oil, in its production, processing, and distribution methods. Reducing carbon emissions and the food system's overall carbon footprint from seed to fork are critical environmental goals, though how to achieve them remains only one of many debates within the movement.

What is less in doubt, and stems partially from the energy-impact debate, is the near-legendary status accorded "local." Whether locally produced and distributed food—and many definitions of "local" abound—staves off the inevitability of global warming, legions of consumers are seeking it out. Their reasons include its positive impact on regional economies, individual health, and the quality of community life. But I want to suggest a significant feature of local that doesn't always find its way into the critique, and that is the notion of intimacy. If true intimacy between two or more people, whether in a family, between lovers and among friends, or with a higher being, is one of the most rewarding of all human experiences, then the intimacy that might exist between a person and nonhuman things—animals, plants, landscapes—may offer similar rewards. "Knowing where your food comes from" has become an unfortunate cliché in the local food movement, but if one is able to use food as a bridge to a richer world of possibilities—nature and the land, gardening, a heritage of farming and ranching, family meals, spiritual and religious practices—then a variety of doors are flung open that can lead to new pathways. I think of something that Charles Kuralt of CBS's *On the Road* fame once said: "Thanks to the interstate highway system, it is now possible to travel from coast to coast without seeing anything." Thanks to the industrial food system, it is now possible to eat whatever we want whenever we want it without having a clue about who produced it or where. Anonymity, that sad beast of modernism, is just one of many Achilles' heels of our industrial food model.

One of the more striking attributes of the alternative food system is that it is not shy about claiming more territory for its own. For instance, the subject of farm animal welfare is no longer the sole province of eccentric humane treatment advocates, some of whom wince at the sight of a swatted fly. Factory farms, confined animal feeding operations, hormone and antibiotic injections, and the numerous accounts of willful abuse and neglect of livestock have driven many consumers into the alternative food system camp and millions more into a life of passionate vegetarianism.

Other territory claimed by alternative food includes the realms of justice and democracy. More specifically, food justice, food democracy, and food sovereignty have entered the lexicon of this colorful movement. Justice and its variations can be summed up by saying that all are entitled to access to healthy and affordable food, and that those who make their living from food—from farmers to busboys—are entitled to wages that allow them to buy healthy food and someday the trappings of a modest middle-class lifestyle.

Democracy and sovereignty are somewhat more nuanced concepts when applied to food. They break into turf previously controlled by free market philosophers. According to our laissez-faire form of capitalism, whose principles still govern most of our economic lives, decisions that affect our food and agriculture system fall unequivocally into the lap of the marketplace. Food democracy and food sovereignty advocates are saying, "Sorry, there's more to it than that. If we are citizens and have the right to vote, and if we are consumers and have the right to eat, then we also have the right to participate in decisions that determine the 'how's' and 'where's' of our food."

Most of the major tenets of the alternative food system have been well organized and defined by the W. K. Kellogg Foundation's Food and Society program. Ricardo Salvador, a foundation program director and agronomist formerly on the faculty at Iowa State University, developed definitions and measurements for food that embodies four characteristics of the alternative food movement. "Good food" is:

1. Healthy—food that is nutritious and readily available; food that over time won't lead to heart disease, diabetes, or other chronic, diet-related problems;
2. Green—produced in an environmentally sustainable manner, but not necessarily organic;
3. Fair—all who are involved in the food system from production to point of purchase receive fair wages and have safe working conditions; no one in the food chain is exploited;
4. Affordable—people have the means to purchase it.

Now, "good food" may not cover all the bases—it's a little ambiguous when it comes to its origins, and "environmentally sustainable" leaves more wiggle room than many people like. Neither is it particular about where good food is sold or how it is distributed. Good food, according to this definition, could be purchased at Wal-Mart as easily as it could at a farmers' market. But the construct offers broad parameters that, at least according to the foundation, are measurable. That ability to actually quantify how much of this food is out there, and more importantly, how many consumers are eating it, is critical for determining the progress of the alternative food system when compared to the industrial food system. And by the measures that have been developed by the foundation as of 2007, 1.8 percent of U.S. food sales was classified as good food. The foundation's hope, one that will be supported by appropriate philanthropy, is to push that number to 10 percent by 2016. This is part of a campaign that has been dubbed "2 to 10."

Related measures of alternative food exist. For instance, there are more farmers' markets, more small farmers, more direct marketing of all descriptions than ever before. Organic food sales are the fastest growing segment of the retail food industry. Virtually every major chain food store, including Wal-Mart, has climbed on board the green train, which has been chugging down the tracks with ever-greater velocity. According to the U.S. Department of Agriculture's 2007 Census of Agriculture, direct food marketing from the farmer to the consumer was valued at just a hair over $1 billion.

Now, as a share of total agricultural sales, that figure is minute, ranging from a high of 3.9 percent of all agricultural sales in the Northeast to a low of 0.4 percent in the Southeast. Most startling, however, are the comparative growth rates. Across the nation, direct sales have grown by 105 percent between 1997 and 2007, compared to only 48 percent for total agricultural sales. These sales are coming from about 136,000 farms, about 6 percent of all U.S. farms, and are in large part the reason that farmers' markets, community-supported agriculture, and farm-to-school programs (along with their variations, including farm-to-college and farm-to-hospital) are expanding by leaps and bounds.

The 2007 agricultural census also found an increase in the number of farms, now 2.2 million, up by 75,810 since 2002. U.S. farm acreage that is certified organic under USDA standards increased from 2 million acres in 2000 to 4 million in 2005. Similarly, the number of livestock raised according to certified organic practices jumped from 3.2 million head in 2000 to 14.2 million in 2005. As a percent of total U.S. food sales, organic went from 1.2 percent in 2000 to 2.5 percent in 2005. It is on track to reach somewhere between 5 and 10 percent by 2010. The biggest jump of all during this five-year period came in the number of organic farms—from 12,000 to 18,000.

The sales of food products that are identified as "locally grown" are also climbing dramatically. According to market research publisher Packaged Facts, sales of locally grown food went from $4 billion annually in 2002 to $5 billion in 2007. Sales of $7 billion are expected by 2011. Keep in mind that this is a measurement of "fresh" sales—mostly produce but some dairy and meat. Total fresh sales in the U.S. were pegged at $230 billion in 2005, with fresh produce surpassing fresh meat as the top-selling fresh food category.

The numbers keep piling up—5,200 farmers' markets in 2009; 1,800 community-supported agriculture farms (some have estimated 2,300); 1,200 school districts that include 9,000 individual schools (about 10 percent of the nation's total) are buying at least some food from local farmers; 333 colleges and universities are buying hundreds of millions of dollars' worth of locally produced food as of 2009.

It's hard to say what's behind this growth in the alternative food system. A 2007 article in *Advertising Age* described the "locavore" movement as nonoppositional, in the sense that it wasn't *against* something, like the industrial food system, more that it was *for* something, like local businesses, Main Street, and local food.

Another recent motivation behind the march to local is certainly food safety. The never-ending list of food product contaminations, investigations, and recalls have sent consumers running for the shelter of something more familiar, more trustworthy, and yes, more intimate. With something in excess of $75 billion worth of food products imported annually from 175 countries, American consumers are growing increasingly nervous about places (and farms) that they can't begin to visualize. And since only 1 percent of that imported food receives a food safety inspection at U.S. points of entry, there is every reason for consumers to be wary.

SO WE'VE WON?

Before we go any further, let's check back with the numbers. A little over 2 percent of food sales are "good food" now, projected to go to only 10 percent by 2016; perhaps 6 percent of all farmers are engaged in direct marketing; there has been a slight uptick in the number of farms but at the same time, according to the American Farmland Trust, a continuing annual loss of 1.2 million acres of farmland; so-called local food sales are around $5 billion, which is barely 2 percent of all fresh food sales in the U.S.; and colleges and universities are responding to student demand for sustainable dining, but only a minority of the nation's schools are participating in the movement, and generally only the more elite (translate as expensive) are sourcing even one-third (definitely the highest estimate among those institutions) of their food from local sources —sustainable or not. What's obvious is that by every measure that counts, with the possible exception of enthusiasm, the alternative food movement has a long way to go. If they were dogs, the "alternatives" would be the intrepid Chihuahua nipping tenaciously at the ankles of the mastiff, the "industrials."

And like prophets proclaiming the coming of the Messiah, the press gushes with unfettered exuberance. Take *Business Week* magazine, which proclaimed, "The rise of farmers' markets . . . is a testament to a dramatic shift in American tastes. . . . [Local food] is reshaping the business of growing and supplying food to Americans. . . . The impact of 'locavores' even shows up in . . . the [2008] Farm Bill [in which] $2.3 billion [out of $290 billion] was set aside for specialty crops" (a rough synonym for local food). Again, enthusiasm has eclipsed the evidence.

Where *Business Week* did get it right is in crediting the giants of food retailing for their growing embrace of local and sustainable food. Many purists in the alternative food movement, of course, look askance at these efforts by mainstream retailers like Wal-Mart and Kroger, and they even have their questions about Whole Foods. One could say that, like the American auto industry that couldn't build a small, energy-efficient car, chain retailers are Johnnies-come-lately to the good food game. At worst, one can say that this is just "greenwashing" and that the retailers are going to display their newfound environmental consciences only as long as they make money from it. Regardless of their motivations, this mainstreaming of "alternative food" into the conventional food system does push food that had previously been the province of the elite into territory more easily reached by everyone.

Whole Foods claims that it is spending 22 percent of its produce budget on locally grown products as of 2008, up from 15 percent four years previously. The company defines as local food that doesn't travel any more than seven hours to the store where it's sold. Wal-Mart's version of local is anything grown within the state where it's sold. According to the consumer research firm the Hartman Group, consumers themselves define as local food that comes from within a 100-mile radius or in-state. This is at least a vast improvement from a day in the late 1990s when the head produce buyer for a major New England supermarket chain told me his definition of local was "anything that I can get from the field to my loading dock in twenty-four hours, including the Chilean grapes that are airfreighted overnight to Logan Airport" in Boston.

Some food retailers, like the $38 billion per year Supervalu chain, are putting products in special containers to give food a homey and local look. At their two Sunflower stores in Columbus, Ohio, the company is selling milk in old-fashioned glass bottles (the label says the milk has traveled 97.3 miles to reach the store). Others are just as assiduously taking things out of their products. Dannon yogurt announced in February 2009 that it would stop using milk made with the rBGH, an artificial growth hormone injected in dairy cows to increase milk production (that the decision was made only two weeks after Yoplait yogurt made the same announcement is, of course, coincidental).

Some food corporations are tripping over each other to burnish their public images with the creation of new staff positions (announced in glowing company press releases) that in some cases make the employer sound more sacred than secular—or at least holier-than-thou. Sodexo, the $7.7 billion per year, 120,000-employee food service company, has a vice president for Corporate Citizenship and one person assigned to its Stop Hunger project, which includes Sodexo Servathon, Feeding Our Future, Community Kitchens, and related food donation programs. To prove finally that they are indeed ethical, some corporations, like Starbucks, which has worked hard to annihilate almost every truly local coffeehouse in America, simply create so-called ethical positions. In 2008 the corporation announced an opening for an "ethical sourcing manager" with a range of duties that include monitoring Starbuck's progress toward a number of yes, ethical objectives. Presumably the unethical sourcing manager is located in a different office.

FOOD CRISIS

How much of this interest in the alternative food movement and its values—whether expressed at farmers' markets or mega-markets—can be sustained in the face of economic pressure is a central question. Two forces have been at work recently that imperil both the global food system and the alternative food system. In June 2009 *National Geographic* magazine devoted an entire issue (labeled the "The Global Food Crisis") to the worldwide food shortages and resulting increase in food prices that have been taking place since 2005. Noting that the price of wheat and corn had tripled over the previous year, the price of rice had climbed fivefold, and that food riots had occurred in two dozen countries, *National Geographic* stated that "the world has been consuming more food than it has been producing." Joachim von Braun, director general of the international Food Policy Research Institute in Washington, DC, was quoted as saying, "Agricultural productivity growth is only one to two percent a year. This is too low to meet population growth and increased demand." Worldwide, food prices rose 75 percent from 2000 to 2007 (according to the Center on International Cooperation), and the *Economist* magazine's food price index was higher in late 2007 than at any time since its creation in 1845.

Though the U.S. food system has far greater resilience than those of developing nations, Americans have nevertheless felt the sting. Food prices jumped as much as 3 percent in one month during 2008, and at least for a while modified consumer purchasing behavior. For example, one Salt Lake City shopper was quoted by the *Deseret News* as saying, "I went grocery shopping . . . and it killed me. I spent $750 . . . and I didn't buy any meat." Her normal monthly food bill had been $650. Sales at Wal-Mart and McDonald's—virtually the low-price leaders in their respective sectors—have been up. In Great Britain, sales of baked beans, reminiscent of postwar rationing years, have increased 12 percent. And in what can only be considered the most accurate barometer of hard times, to say nothing of how low one can go, Spam sales in the U.S. were up more than 10 percent.

While hard times for the poor and near poor are nothing new, the food stamp program was at record participation levels—about 37 million Americans as of December 2009—and food banks were unable to keep up with demand. Emergency food sites across the nation were experiencing requests two to three times above their normal levels and were forced to dig deeper into food stocks that were not being replenished by their equally stressed donors. For the poor there is the compounding effect of economic pressure, rising food prices, and public subsidies and charitable donations that don't keep pace with need. Healthier food that costs more, such as fresh fruits and vegetables, is replaced by high-calorie junk food, like soda and fatty snacks, which drives up obesity levels, especially for the poor. A 2008 study by the U.S. Department of Health and Human Services found that women in poverty were roughly 50 percent more likely to be obese than those with higher socioeconomic status.

School food service directors ("lunch ladies") must cut back on food quality since they are required to live within fixed budgets established by federal reimbursements. Typically these reimbursement rates are adjusted only periodically and will lag behind actual food costs, especially in times of inflation. In response to shrinking budgets and soaring growth in free and reduced-price meals, cafeteria workers in the Albuquerque, New Mexico, school district resorted to making cheese sandwiches from surplus commodity cheese for hungry kids.

A number of factors are at play. Rising food prices are due to rising energy prices, a switch in agricultural acreage away from food crops to biofuel crops, drought in some parts of the world (Australia), and growing demand for meat among populations that previously ate little of that item (per person, the Chinese now eat 110 pounds of meat annually compared to 44 pounds in 1985). But even when food prices moderated and began to drop in 2009, the global economic downturn sent many people to the unemployment line, which forced another round of belt tightening and the pursuit, again, of cheap food. Even some elite shoppers are descending from the towering heights of high-end farmers' markets, seeking relief from $9-a-pound organic chicken and $5-a-pound tomatoes in the aisles of the more prosaic Trader Joe's.

Price spikes come and price spikes go. Throughout the ages there has been a long history of frequent disruptions in food production, occasionally resulting in shortages, riots, rebellions, and even coups d'état. Things, however, have a way of returning to normal, of seeking a balance or a new level, whether through government intervention, international relief efforts, human migration, or, in the most extreme Malthusian response, populations dying off in proportion to available food stocks.

But the question of our food future remains, and perhaps this time with more urgency than in days gone by. Paul Roberts in *The End of Food* asks not just "whether we'll be able to feed 9.5 billion people by 2050," but "how long we can continue to meet the demands of the 6.5 billion alive today." Population growth is approaching unsustainable levels, now certainly in the teeming cities of the developing world, and elsewhere by the mid-twenty-first century. Not only does this give us more hungry mouths to feed, but competing needs for nonagricultural land use will reduce the arable land base necessary for food production. The rush from agrarianism to urbanism has stripped away our land base, farming skills, and, perhaps most profoundly, a primal unity between humanity and nature.

There is no doubt that the climate is changing and that the impact on future growing conditions in different parts of the world is far from known. With increasing investments required to produce food, the last thing a farmer needs is more unpredictability. Humankind's expanding skill in unraveling the secrets of nature and applying that knowledge to the needs at hand has taken more of us from barely understanding how "it" works into the realms of the utterly incomprehensible.

This mastery of science by a priesthood shrinking in numbers in proportion to the general population is as powerful as it is risky. When institutional food production, technology, financial incentive and distribution power are placed in the hands of the few; when corporate might and the pull of money set the agenda, we feel control of our food system slipping away and our tenuous grip on democracy loosening. Do we trade in a hands-on role in our food system for the promise we'll be fed by others? Do we forfeit our intellect, our passion, and the muscles and tendons of our arms for the peace that comes from knowing that food will be provided? Do we mute our voices and let others who claim a higher wisdom in these matters make the decisions for us? These may very well be the questions we must find answers to, questions that are even bigger than how we feed a hungry world. Finding ways to reassert our control in the face of power, to relearn skills that have atrophied during ages of dependency and neglect, and to rediscover a triumphant kind individualism that embraces both the self and community are the tasks that confront twenty-first-century adherents of the alternative food system.

THE GRAND INQUISITOR

As I look into the future of food and democracy in the twenty-first century, I see two options: we will either shape our own food destiny or we will succumb to one that is presented to us. Placing ourselves in the hands of others can be either an act of profound trust or one of unsettling risk. Yet the question may not be answered solely by the relative merits of either choice—would I prefer a food system I direct and manage myself to one that is managed by others?—nor should it necessarily be based on the degree of risk one is willing to accept. The answer to the question may in fact turn on more humanistic considerations, such as how can we live more intimately, more profoundly, and more vividly? These values enter the equation when we choose to pursue the alternative food system rather than be pursued by the industrial food system. The consequences of either choice go beyond the possible biological and economic impacts, although of course these do matter, and may speak most immediately to what is best for the human soul.

For some guidance on how to understand this question, let's go back for a moment to the nineteenth century. Though there may not be many Dostoevskians among those who ponder the future of food, I found it instructive to look at a parable that appears in the Russian novel *The Brothers Karamazov,* completed in 1880, perhaps the greatest achievement of Fyodor Dostoevsky, one of Western literature's supreme novelists.

The parable is called "The Grand Inquisitor" and occupies a mere 19 pages in the hefty 770-page volume. Though the parable is the product of Dostoevsky's prodigious literary imagination, its import transcends the expected interest of literary scholars and has fascinated political scientists, theologians, philosophers, and psychologists across three centuries. No less a cultural icon than Sigmund Freud considered *The Brothers Karamazov* the greatest novel ever written, and "The Grand Inquisitor" "one of the peaks in the literature of the world."

The novel depicts a grand struggle within the Karamazov clan, but at a broader level concerns itself with what one of the brothers, Ivan Karamazov, calls "the eternal questions, of the existence of God and immortality." As another brother, Dmitri, puts it, "God and the devil are fighting . . . and the battlefield is the heart of man."

The story is set in sixteenth-century Spain at the height of the Spanish Inquisition. Jesus Christ appears on the plaza the day after 100 "heretics" have been publicly burned by the cardinal. The Grand Inquisitor, recognizing Jesus as a threat to his authority, has Him arrested and sentences Him to be burned the following day. When the Inquisitor visits Christ in His cell, their conversation centers on whether freedom is a gift to humankind or a burden it's better relieved of.

The Grand Inquisitor berates Christ for doing a great disservice to humanity by not taking up the devil's temptation to turn stones into bread and water into wine. Instead, Christ chose to persuade humanity that it was free to follow His teachings without Him resorting to miracles. The Grand Inquisitor decries this approach, asserting that people are too weak, and that "nothing has ever been more insupportable for man than freedom. . . . Turn [stones] into bread, and mankind will run after Thee like a flock of sheep, grateful and obedient. . . . But Thou would not deprive man of freedom and did reject the offer, thinking, what is that freedom worth, if obedience is bought with bread?"

In his cynical certainty, the Inquisitor believes that he is the ultimate authority to which humankind will submit once he has guaranteed the people bread, and again chastises Christ for His naïveté. "There is no crime, and therefore no sin; there is only hunger. Feed men, and then ask of them virtue! . . . They will find us and cry to us, 'Feed us.' Oh, never, never can they feed themselves without us! No science will give them bread so long as they remain free. In the end they will lay their freedom at our feet, and say to us, 'Make us your slaves, but feed us.'"

The Inquisitor acknowledges that some have chosen to follow

Christ freely, without the benefit of contrivances or false submission. While that might be fine for that relatively small percentage of humankind, he accuses Christ of turning His back on the vast majority who might be left to face certain starvation. "And for the sake of the bread of heaven tens of thousands shall follow Thee, but what is to become of the millions and tens of millions of creatures who will not have the strength to forego the earthly bread for the sake of the heavenly? No, we care for the weak too. . . . give bread, and man will worship thee, for nothing is more certain than bread."

Again, the Inquisitor contemptuously criticizes Christ for His rejection of the three powers that hold humankind in their sway: "those forces are miracle, mystery, and authority. . . . Is the nature of men such, that they can reject miracle? . . . for man seeks not so much God as the miraculous. And as man cannot bear to be without the miraculous, he will worship deeds of sorcery and witchcraft."

Christ says not a word during this one-way interrogation. This makes the Inquisitor anxious, since he has assumed that Christ will offer some embittered defense. Instead, Christ looks gently into the old man's face and silently rises to place a kiss on the Inquisitor's "bloodless aged lips. That was all His answer. The old man shuddered. . . . He went to the door, opened it, and said to Him: 'Go, and come no more.' And he let Him out into the dark alleys of the town." Christ is free and the Grand Inquisitor is shaken.

Did Christ or the Grand Inquisitor win the debate? Before jumping too readily to Christ's side and castigating the evil incarnate embodied by the Grand Inquisitor, consider that Dostoevsky, and numerous commentators and scholars have called it a draw or found in favor of the Cardinal. As the scholar Jerry S. Wasserman has written, "[M]uch of the difficulty—and the greatness—of 'The Grand Inquisitor' arises from the fact that Christ does not clearly triumph. . . . [Dostoevsky] never succeeded in convincing himself that he had adequately disputed the powerful poison logic of the Grand Inquisitor. A respectable number of critics and commentators share Dostoevsky's doubts."

Who can claim that humankind is not weak and has not descended on occasion to the most degrading depth when faced with an extreme crisis such as hunger? (One example: Protestant soup kitchens sprang up in Catholic areas during the Irish potato famine. "Taking the soup" became slang for giving up your values in exchange for gain.) How proud will humankind be when faced with the choice between clinging stubbornly to freedom—whether granted by a higher being or through individual instinct—or avoiding starvation? If authority—whether in the form of a government, a food industry, or even a charitable foundation—offers what we perceive to be an answer to a very difficult problem that threatens large numbers of us, and all that is required is that we submit to that authority, what might be the lesser of two evils? And when solutions are offered that are based on supposedly irrefutable science (developed and managed by humans, of course, but still largely a mystery to most of us) and that, we are told by the experts, have the power to improve the quality of our lives, do we even raise the possibility that we may not want them?

Millions are now following a path of thoughtful independence in order to be free of the industrial food system. They are faithful to the notion that they can achieve healthier lifestyles, cleanse the planet, and bring a more profound form of human intimacy to their lives by pursuing a different kind of food system. Billions, on the other hand, have little problem with the industrial food system and little interest in the alternative. Whether by accident of circumstance or the design of authority figures, the great mass of humanity sees no higher purpose served in pursuing a different kind of food system. The one that is readily available and controlled by a relatively few number of people, agencies, and corporations seems perfectly adequate.

Who is winning the debate now between Christ and the Grand Inquisitor is an important question, but who will win it in the years to come is even more critical because it will determine *who determines* the future of our food, and more profoundly, the future of humankind. Will we eat the heavenly bread or the earthly bread?

CHAPTER 3

THE INDUSTRIAL FOOD SYSTEM
Ministry of Plenty or Department of Destruction?

While there can be little doubt that never have so few produced so much food for so many, such abundance has come at a high cost to the environment, human health, food and agricultural workers, farm animals, wildlife, and the social and economic fabric of many American communities. Of course, that harm has not occurred everywhere, or all the time. There are indeed many good, clean, and responsible operators within the system. But there can be little question now that grievous sins have been committed and that the threat to the future is genuine.

I don't wish to restate the long litany of damage here—volumes on that subject already exist—but only to provide a few examples of how the industrial food system has worked its will on the planet and its people. The larger question we face is whether the industrial food system can reform itself. Should we give it a shot at redemption and hope that the positive examples of a few major food system players are indeed harbingers of a new paradigm? Even for those attempting to "get right with their Lord," we still must ask if the spirit of the Grand Inquisitor is not close to their hearts.

CONVENTIONAL AND FACTORY FARMING
Conventional agriculture (nonorganic and not making comprehensive use of sustainable farming practices) relies heavily on agricultural chemicals for fertilizer, pesticides, herbicides, and fungicides. One class of pesticides, organophosphates, is made from chemicals

derived from World War II–era nerve gases and can damage the mental and physical development of infants and children. Because of their inherent risk, scientists and environmental regulators have requested that the federal government ban twenty organophosphate pesticides. Under the administration of George W. Bush, however, the Environmental Protection Agency (EPA), which has jurisdiction over such matters, permitted the continued use of most of these. In major growing regions of the western United States, such as California's Central Valley, much of Washington State, Oregon, and southern Arizona, the use of these harmful chemicals to grow the vast majority of America's fresh food supply continues.

Factory farms, also known as confined animal feeding operations (CAFOs), have eclipsed pesticide use in the public's eye as the most egregious offender in the industrial food system. Whether the land is used for raising dairy cows, beef cattle, poultry, or hogs, major sections of the United States have been "colonized" by these farms and their related operations (cheese-processing facilities, slaughter- and packinghouses), and they are massive in scale. In the eleven states of the western region, there are well over 2000 CAFOs. If one moves east into Texas, one sees enormous numbers of factory dairy and cattle farms; such towns as Hereford and Amarillo suffocate under a hazy pall of stagnant air, feedlot dust, and manure odors. Hogs rule in the Oklahoma Panhandle, where the Kerr Center has documented the decimating effect that industry has had on community life, employment, and the environment, aided and abetted by a local and state political system that's willing to accept any industry that promises jobs. From Maryland south to North Carolina and Georgia, poultry and hog CAFOs have destroyed waterways, exploited workers (mostly immigrants), and created havoc with air quality.

While these operations are responsible for an array of outrageous abuses to people and animals, even worse are their environmental impacts, specifically in the form of air and water damage. Since CAFOs produce ungodly quantities of manure (each dairy cow, for instance, produces four tons of manure per year; one 5,000-head dairy CAFO produces as much excrement as a small city), the primary threat to the environment is in the form of nitrates percolating into both surface water and groundwater. Generally, the amount of seepage into the water supply is controlled by waste management permits granted by EPA and state environmental agencies. But the operative word here is "permit." Pollution, up to a certain amount, is permitted; anything beyond certain levels (in the case of nitrates, no more than ten parts per million), constitutes a violation. In New Mexico, which has 300,000 dairy cows that produce enough manure each day to fill up nine Olympic-size swimming pools, two-thirds of the state's 150 dairy CAFOs are in violation of permitted groundwater nitrate levels. And given the process of environmental monitoring and enforcement, it can take years (some are convinced it will never happen) for the state regulators to stop the pollution and force the perpetrators to clean up.

In the meantime, residents of dairy CAFO communities endure enormous hardships. Families are unable to have outdoor picnics in the warm weather because the flies are on the food before the Saran Wrap can be removed from the potato salad. One resident of eastern New Mexico told me that the entire south-facing outside wall of his house, normally light-colored stucco, becomes black with flies at certain times of the year. Even though he kills them with an insecticide one day, they are back the next. Groundwater tables have dropped so low due to the high water usage of CAFOs that homeowners must drill their wells deeper at considerable expense, not only for the drilling but also for the higher energy costs associated with pumping water a greater distance. Concern about groundwater contamination has also driven many residents to buy bottled water. Air pollution, which is monitored only sporadically in some parts of New Mexico, is also associated with asthma rates, which tend to run significantly higher in the state's dairy regions.

CAFOs have been responsible for ruining some of the nation's most scenic and ecologically rich waterways. In Maryland, the poultry industry went from 90 million chickens in 1960 to 270 million in 2005. As reported in the *New York Times,* this threefold growth also resulted in a near tripling of chicken manure generated, to 297,000 tons a year, which is largely responsible for the growth of phosphorous and nitrogen levels in the Chesapeake Bay. This pollution caused the number of oystermen who worked the bay to drop from 6,000 to fewer than 500. The heritage Chesapeake blue crab population has plummeted by 70 percent. Yes, chicken factories have succeeded in producing a skinless chicken breast for less than $2 per pound retail, but they have taken down the region's seafood industry and probably some portion of the Chesapeake's tourist industry at the same time. After all, who wants to go boating in the pea-green soup caused by farming's nutrient-generated algae blooms?

As the toll mounts from factory livestock production, we see the risk to the public health change from things we can see, smell, or taste (our senses having always been our best defense against danger) to things that are not easily detectable, things that couldn't even be imagined many years ago. Human resistance to antibiotics is one such threat. A particular strain of bacteria that, according to the *Journal of the American Medical Association,* is responsible for 19,000 deaths a year in the United States—that's more than AIDS kills—is winning the war against antibiotics. The widespread nontherapeutic use of antibiotics (using them routinely on livestock as a preventative measure in factory farm situations where the risk of infection is high because animals are so tightly confined) is suspected as a culprit in the skyrocketing number of antibiotic resistance cases in humans. This seems probable given that the Union of Concerned Scientists estimates that at least 70 percent of the antibiotics used in America are fed to livestock on factory farms. Fortunately, the Obama administration is seeking a ban on antibiotic use in farm animals unless it is for the treatment of specific illnesses and done under the supervision of a veterinarian. It can be assumed that the livestock industry will fight the proposed ban, and should it lose the fight now will most likely resume the fight once the political winds shift again.

America's medical community has also spoken out against factory livestock farming. The American Public Health Association called for a moratorium on the development of all future CAFOs until a series of environmental, health, and social issues could be scientifically addressed and resolved. In 2006 the Pew Charitable Trusts convened a commission on industrial farm animal production. This commission issued a report in 2008 recommending new laws regulating pollution from industrial farms, a phasing-out of CAFOs that restrict "natural movement and normal behavior," a ban on hormones to promote animal growth, and an application of antitrust laws to encourage more competition and less concentration in the livestock industry.

FARM WORKERS

One part of the industrial food story that doesn't receive much attention is the plight of food and farm workers. Like any factory system that is designed to produce large quantities of products in a uniform manner, industrial farming requires large numbers of workers performing rote tasks under stressful and often dangerous working conditions. Like any industry that is dominated by capital and only minimally regulated, the wages paid to labor will be as low as possible. In the case of farming, wages are rarely adequate to meet even the minimum standard of a middle-class lifestyle. And it's not only the large industrial food players who play fast and loose with labor; the organic food industry is often culpable as well. Remember, to qualify for good food status, it's not enough to produce food with "green" or sustainable farming methods, the food must also be produced fairly, which means using nonexploitive labor practices. Irv Hershenbaum, a United Farm Workers union leader, noted in an article (posted on Alternet) that organic farm workers may not be exposed to pesticides, but like workers on conventional farms they go without many of the basic protections that are taken for granted in other blue-collar industries.

In one of the more publicly exposed examples of both worker and animal abuse (it's questionable if many industrial food operators would recognize the difference), Agriprocessors, Inc., one of the nation's largest kosher meatpackers, was fined $10 million by the state of Iowa for labor violations, including 9,311 criminal misdemeanor charges concerning child labor laws. Similarly, the animal rights organization People for the Ethical Treatment of Animals (PETA) recorded numerous acts of inhumane treatment of animals at the same meatpacking plant when one of their members went undercover for seven weeks and filmed those abuses. According to the *New York Times,* this "prompted the U.S. Department of Agriculture to conduct a six-month investigation, which reported many violations of animal cruelty laws at the plant." The violations of both human and animal dignity were so extreme that the Orthodox Union, the major kosher certifying organization in the United States, called for Agriprocessors' kosher decertification unless substantial changes were made.

Sectors of the industrial food system may rightfully invoke the "one bad apple doesn't ruin the whole bunch" adage with respect to the behavior of some of its individual members. Likewise, in any group of baseball players, there will always be a few who use steroids, cork their bats, or throw spitballs. It goes with the territory and that's why we have rules and umpires. You get caught, you get thrown out. The larger integrity of the team and the sport are preserved.

But there could very well be something about the moral framework of the industrial food system that its members feel allows them to transcend the rules of conduct that most of us live by. Perhaps it's a sense of entitlement that comes from believing that they are feeding a hungry world, or that their association with farming, food distribution, or some aspect of the agro-technology complex means they are not subject to the rules that govern the rest of civilized society. In this state of mind, purveyors of and apologists for agro-science display a kind of chilly arrogance; seemingly they have come to regard ordinary people as dependent on their sacred knowledge for survival. Furthermore, they often take as gospel the belief that nonfarmers have no right to challenge the dominant food system.

INDUSTRIAL FARMING ARROGANCE, THE NEW MEXICO WAY

The scene was set for one more act of agricultural hubris in Room 309 of the New Mexico state capitol on February 17, 2009. The state's antipoverty and social justice organizations had brought a bill before the state legislature to require that all but the smallest of the state's farms and ranches provide workers' compensation coverage for their nonfamily employees. Workers' compensation is a form of insurance that pays for the cost of treating work-related injuries. It is "experience related," which means that the more claims and medical payouts that are made, the more expensive the insurance premiums will be. Since farming and ranching are considered risky occupations, insurance premiums are considerably higher on average than they are for, say, computer programmers. All states are required by their respective laws to provide workers' compensation coverage for all occupations—with one exception. In eight states, including New Mexico, all agricultural occupations are exempt from mandatory workers' compensation coverage. Not mining, not law enforcement, not alligator wrestling; only agricultural occupations are exempt. Ironically, this practice, along with other exemptions from various provisions of minimum wage laws, certain child labor practices, and safety and hazard regulations, is a legacy of family-scale farming. With some justification, policy makers have sought to insulate smaller businesses, particularly farms operated only by family members, from what many regard as the more burdensome improvements in America's labor standards. But the industrial food system, invoking the mythology of the family farm and the vestiges of rural self-reliance, sought to codify these exemptions by extending them to large, capital-intensive agribusinesses.

I remember when I first discovered the workers' compensation exemption in the course of reporting on the state's dairy industry. When a New Mexico dairyman told me his industry was not required to provide that coverage, I asked what happened when a worker was injured on the job. He told me that he drops the worker off at the emergency room of the local hospital, which is required by law to treat the injury. The hospital presents a bill to the worker who, as everybody knows perfectly well, can't and won't pay it, then tries to collect from the dairyman. The dairyman told me that he routinely offers to pay the hospital half the cost of treating the injury. Since the hospital is over a barrel, it accepts the dairyman's offer and eats the rest, a loss that is actually assumed at that point by the taxpayer. By industry standards, my dairyman's actions are considered generous, even though his dairy didn't provide workers' compensation insurance and had possibly left the injured worker in the position of not being able to seek additional treatment should it be required.

Back in Room 309, 150 people had crowded into a space that could seat 80. Space was at such a premium that people who were forced to stand guarded their one or two square feet of floor space with a wide stance and extended elbows. When I made the mistake of momentarily leaving my allotted territory to assist a handicapped man struggling to open the hearing room's doors, a short but tough female lobbyist from the New Mexico Farm Bureau bullied her way into my spot and glared at me when I foolishly attempted to retake it. I spent the rest of the hearing pinned against the back wall.

On the right-hand side of the room (both physically and politically) sat the industrial food system—representatives of the state's cattle ranchers' association, Farm Bureau, chile growers' association, dairy producers' association, and even the vineyard growers' association. In violation of the code of the West, the ranchers in the front of the visitors' area refused to remove their cowboy hats, thus deliberately obscuring the view of those in the back. Bolo-tied, slim-waisted, broad-shouldered, and deeply tanned, they seemed to emanate a collective glare that could stop an angry bull. On the left sat the antipoverty advocates, representatives of the Catholic archdiocese, farm workers, small farmers with the state's acequia association, and some public interest attorneys. Unlike their male industrial agricultural counterparts, who invariably had close-cropped haircuts, the "liberals" sported bald heads or bushy, salt-and-pepper coifs. Rather than scowling, their faces were amiable, though etched with lines of concern.

When the chair of the House Labor and Human Resources Committee opened the floor for public comment, it was immediately clear whose oxen would be gored by mandatory workers' compensation coverage. A lobbyist for Dairy Farmers of America, the nation's biggest dairy organization, said the cost of the insurance would add too much to New Mexico's dairy industry's payroll (he neglected to say that the average dairy worker's wage was in the range of $8 to $10 per hour). One well-dressed cattle rancher, whose custom-made boots alone were worth as much as the workers' comp premiums he might have paid for his ranch hands, said that the average net farmer/rancher income in New Mexico was only $19,000. The chile association said that the state's chile production acreage had declined from 36,000 acres to 8,000, and that labor was 60 percent of their costs. "Workmen's compensation coverage would drive many farms out of business," he said, leaving out the part about competition from Mexico being the chief cause of this iconic New Mexico industry's decline. Even the wine growers, who cater to the state's higher-end consumers and tourists, argued against the bill, citing higher costs that they certainly couldn't be expected to absorb.

The pro–workers' comp side had its own ox story to tell, but in their case it was a farm worker who had actually been gored by one. Because of his broken ribs and inability to afford adequate medical treatment (his employer offered to pay nothing), he had been in so much pain he'd been unable to work for two years. One woman said, "Farm workers do cry. Some get fired when they are hurt. Why should farm workers, who are the poorest paid part of agriculture, have to pay when they are hurt on the job?" A representative of the Catholic archdiocese put forward the simple proposition: "A society is judged by how it treats its most vulnerable people. Denying farm workers workmen's compensation violates the common good." A beautiful young Mexican woman, surrounded by hard-looking cowboys, said firmly to the legislators, "This [bill] is a matter of human rights. Human life is not a commodity." An attorney who represents injured workers said that the bill would affect only 7 percent of all farms and ranches in New Mexico, but that would represent 80 percent of all uninsured farm workers, a number estimated at 10,000 people.

In response to the whiny liberals, one Republican member of the committee referred to agriculture as the "Holy Grail" of New Mexico. He said, "Anything that might violate their [agriculture companies'] needs must be taken seriously." In other words, agriculture should not be expected to pay the less than 1 percent of the $2 billion it generates in income each year in New Mexico for the estimated additional cost of workers' compensation. The same legislator went on for nearly thirty minutes interrogating the staff of the lead pro-coverage advocacy organization about its nonprofit status, the source of its funding, and the possible legal and tax implications for violating federal and state laws governing its advocacy work and use of public funds. It was a blatant attempt to disparage the organization's standing before the legislature.

As it has done countless times across the country, Big Ag carried the day in New Mexico. By a vote of 7 to 3 (three Democrats voted with four Republicans), the committee killed the bill. Again, the industrial food system had persuaded policy makers that it should be granted privileges to which no other industry is entitled. Exemption from laws and regulations that govern everyone else is indeed an unrecognized public subsidy—never, of course, to be acknowledged by the industry or its lapdog policy makers.

And for the losers, well, they were the taxpayers, who pick up the costs when agriculture doesn't, and of course the uninsured worker, who patches himself up in the best way he can after an injury so that he can once again place himself at risk to produce our food.

THE INDUSTRIAL FOOD SYSTEM PUTS ON THE GREEN

The industrial food system is working overtime to conform to growing consumer interest in sustainability, and to a lesser extent, social justice. As reported in the *Washington Post*, the Mars candy bar company announced that all of its chocolate products would come from sustainable sources by 2020. Announcements like these always have the tone of altruism about them until you discover the real motives behind them. In this case it is because Mars's competitor, Cadbury, would soon be sporting a fair trade label. Mars also said it would be working with cocoa farmers in Africa to improve their sustainable farming skills in order, of course, to ensure a long-term source of sustainably produced chocolate. But as Paul Rice, chief executive of TransFair USA, which certifies fair trade products, pointed out, "[W]e hope Mars will also take a look at . . . cocoa farmer protection by ensuring that they receive fair wages . . . and fair prices for their crops." Big Food increasingly tells its customers that it is or will produce and/or process its products sustainably because that's what a growing number of its customers want. Working conditions and wages are not necessarily among the top concerns of consumers and therefore receive short shrift.

Along with playing the sustainability card, major food corporations are also offering to reduce pesticides in the food they produce by striking deals with their food suppliers. One of the more recent examples is the McDonald's Corporation consenting to a shareholder resolution brought by Bard College and the AFL-CIO Reserve Fund to conduct a survey of the practices of the company's potato growers. As the largest buyer of potatoes in the U.S., McDonald's is in a position to influence the way that spuds are grown. The survey will determine what those practices are and determine how best to reduce the use of pesticides. Apparently McDonald's is following in the footsteps of the Sysco Corporation, General Mills, and Campbell's, all of which have taken similar action. Holding aside important questions about the objectivity of such studies or what these corporations will actually do with the findings, one might ask why we have so many McDonald's restaurants in the first place, why they resist consumer information strategies such as menu labeling, and why it is necessary for them to dominate so many features of global life. In other words, securing their consent to buy more sustainably produced potatoes might have some short-term benefits, but their dominance over contemporary life remains as strong as ever.

MESSING WITH OUR GENES

Where the industrial food system really seeks to ingratiate itself with public opinion is in the field of biotechnology, particularly with respect to genetically modified organisms (GMOs) used for food. According to the USDA's Economic Research Service, "U.S. farmers have adopted genetically engineered crops widely since their introduction in 1996, notwithstanding uncertainty about consumer acceptance and economic and environmental impacts." In other words, biotech corporations like Monsanto have gone hell for leather to convert American farming to genetically modified seed usage before anyone had the time to consider the long-term consequences, and without consumers having the means, i.e., labeling, to know that they were consuming GMO food. As of 2008 the Economic Research Service reported that 90 percent of all soybean acreage in the U.S. is planted with genetically engineered crops, as are 60 percent of cotton and 55 percent of corn acreage.

Now, to justify its further expansion of GMO crops, particularly in overseas markets, the biotech industry has propagated the myth that only it, and it alone, can feed the world's bourgeoning population (note the Archer Daniel Midland (ADM) company's much-used advertising slogan "Supermarket to the World"). Not only have corporations developed safe technology for that purpose, so they claim, but they also have a moral imperative to use it. In a *Newsweek* opinion piece, Mike Mack, the CEO of Syngenta, a major biotech firm, argued, "Politicians should embrace the potential of science to create a new green revolution. . . . Recession and environmental stresses are deepening existing fears. . . . With technology and global collaboration, farmers around the world can feed the growing population." He went on to castigate the European Union, where "the use of biotechnology in crops has still not been accepted and further constraints are being placed on farmers' ability to use yield-enhancing crop-protection products." Yes, it's true, through their democratic processes, including education, debate, and the transparent workings of government, the people of the European Union have not "accepted" GMO crops. In the United States, we never had a chance to choose. Industry thrust the technology down our throats and has maintained a sustained campaign to secure our acceptance *after the fact.* Knowing that it couldn't use the argument that biotech crops were necessary to feed the U.S., it has disingenuously used that argument to convince the wider world that GMOs are the only path to human survival, implying all the time that those who reject them are ignorant, selfish, or hopelessly idealistic.

The ignorance argument is a particularly interesting one because it is often said by advocates on all sides of food debates that if only consumers really knew the facts, they would most certainly see things "our way." According to Mack, "The public needs to be better informed." This is certainly true, so why didn't the industry, government agencies, and universities offer a national public forum designed to inform the educated layperson of the arguments—pro and con. Perhaps because the industry knew what the answer might have been, or it simply couldn't wait to reap the vast returns from the huge investments in corporate research laboratories. As Mack said, "Syngenta and other leading companies [presumably biotech] spend some $3 billion every year on agricultural research." Shareholders will only wait so long for that research to pay off. And for the industry, that investment finally is. In January 2009 Monsanto announced that its first-quarter net income was $556 million, up from $256 million the year before. The company credited strong expansion into Latin American countries as well as continued growth in U.S. acreage going into GMO seed. Though it reported a $233 million net loss for the final quarter of its 2009 fiscal year, it still ended the fiscal year with a robust $2.1 billion net profit.

To make its case even after the genie has been released from the bottle, the biotech food industry has shrouded itself in a veil of legitimacy and moral certitude by enlisting academics, politicians, and foundation leaders for its cause. Dr. Robert Paarlberg, a political science professor at Wellesley College, wrote *Starved for Science: How Biotechnology is Being Kept out of Africa,* a scathing indictment of the European Union, nongovernment organizations, and some African leaders. He accuses them of preventing the introduction of GMO seed into hungry African nations, saying essentially that they are or will be responsible for mass starvation. The book's foreword is written by Nobel Laureate Norman E. Borlaug and former president Jimmy Carter, both strong advocates for GMO seed. Speaking at Tufts University in the spring of 2009, Paarlberg took a position in favor of very capital-intensive forms of sustainable agriculture that rely on such expensive water- and nutrient-conserving techniques as the laser leveling of agricultural fields. This and the reliance on large tractors and other expensive farm machinery can conserve natural resources, but their cost-effective implementation, by Paarlberg's own admission, requires consolidation of farms into fewer and larger units of operation. Fewer farms, more concentration, more corporate control, and more domination of the food supply by fewer interests lead to adaptation of high-technology solutions—including use of GMO— to the world's food crisis.

In an example of how academia and industry often cohabitate, the *Lincoln Journal Star* reported on the appointment of David Chicoine, president of South Dakota State University, to the eleven-person Monsanto board of directors. The corporation donates millions to land grant universities, which do the bulk of the academic-based agro-research in this county, and South Dakota State has received hundreds of thousands of dollars from Monsanto. Chicoine, an agricultural economist by training, will be paid $195,000 per year in director's fees and a like amount in stock. Not bad for a guy who is making only $300,000 in annual salary as a university president.

But it's in the world of philanthropy that we see even stranger bedfellows. The Bill and Melinda Gates Foundation announced a gift of $5.7 million to the Donald Danforth Plant Science Center to secure the approval of African governments for field-testing of genetically modified crops. Big foundation money is apparently needed to make governments see what they apparently fail to realize is in their best interest. Perhaps this is part of what Syngenta's Mack was referring to when he said that the public must be better informed.

As Katha Pollit pointed out in the *Nation*, "Bill Gates, George Soros, and other titans became masters of a burgeoning nonprofit universe, donating huge sums for healthcare, education, [and] antipoverty programs." In effect, a handful of "titans," whether assembled on Mount Olympus or in Davos, are making "public" policy in a very private way. Their interventions over time will determine society's winners and losers, who controls science and technology, and how resources will be allocated. How did this happen? How did the privilege of making public policy, normally a right only of the people and their elected representatives, devolve to a self-anointed priesthood of extraordinarily rich people? Pollit offers part of the reason. "The boom in philanthropy paralleled—and helped justify—tax cuts, shrunken government services and rising inequality." Government, in other words, our collective expression of democracy in action, was denied the financial resources that instead accumulated disproportionately with a growing band of plutocrats. And when government can't and/or won't act, those who are motivated by their individual sense of what's right and who are not accountable to anyone but themselves become the policy makers. This appears to be the case in the surging movement to bring GMOs to the entire planet, whether or not ordinary citizens understand them or want them.

A great celebration of the elite world food network was held in Des Moines, Iowa, in October 2009 to bestow the World Food Prize. The event, titled Food, Agriculture and National Security in a Globalized World, featured Bill Gates, Ellen Kullman (CEO, Dupont), Indra Nooyi (CEO, PepsiCo), Patricia Woertz (CEO, Archer Daniels Midland), Gene Kahn (VP, General Mills), and Vicki Escarra (CEO, Feeding America). (Dr. Normal Borlaug, also slated to attend, passed away only days before the event.) The corporate, charitable, and foundation leaders gathered to "participate in compelling conversations on topics related to enhancing food security."

In all fairness I should say that I was invited to attend the event, but graciously declined. Not only was the price tag a bit steep, I was worried that I might sully my reputation by being seen with that crowd. More to the point, there is something that makes me nervous when people view serious social and economic problems from the top down. After they have made their fortunes and garnered as much power as their corporate and political ties will allow, they now turn in the spirit of noblesse oblige to address the downtrodden of the earth. Their patience with the world of public policy, governments, and the noisy rabble that is the people is minimal. They have the means, the connections, and the business acumen to avoid it, so why engage with the messy sausage making that is democracy and public policy? And if they can put a few more dollars in the pockets of hardworking agro-corporations along the way, and indeed strengthen the ability of those corporations to exercise even greater control, then why not? In the long run, engaging philanthropy as a partner to agribusiness will only protect, expand, and enhance their influence in proportion to the growth in corporate power.

THE INDUSTRIAL FOOD SYSTEM ON THE OFFENSIVE

Those are some of the more benign and occasionally beneficial behaviors of the industrial food system. Whether its actions are taken out of a genuine interest in "doing good" or are a slick form of "greenwashing" is less important than its ability to make us *believe* that it has our best interests at heart. It is in its own public pronouncements that we might discover the true intent of the industrial food system, and these suggest that it may indeed prefer dominance to fairness and authority to freedom.

There are at least four significant ways in which the industrial food system is unambiguously fighting for control of more territory: framing the issues in ways that make it appear either to be doing good or at least doing no harm; undermining democracy through legislative and legal actions; taking its business "offshore" by expanding into new foreign markets; and painting the alternative food system as an inadequate answer to world food needs.

Perhaps the best discussion to date on how the industrial food system is framing the debate was provided recently in an essay by Kelly Brownell and Kenneth Warner, of Yale University and the University of Michigan respectively. The authors compare Big Tobacco's decades-long effort to avoid responsibility for millions of tobacco-related deaths to the manner in which Big Food tries to avoid responsibility for obesity and diet-related problems. Much of the framing battle revolves around the question of personal responsibility versus industry or societal responsibility. If Big Food (or Big Tobacco) can prove that harmful behavior (eating too much junk food or smoking too many cigarettes) is the fault of individuals because they are undisciplined, ignorant, or otherwise flawed, then they can effectively escape responsibility for producing and distributing unhealthy products. If the proof goes the other way, that Big Food is culpable in manipulating the public (for example, designing ads for sugary soft drinks that target children or locating fast food joints near public schools), then government can be justified in intervening on behalf of the consumer and possibly regulating Big Food. As the authors make clear, "These points [made by Big Food] play well in America—personal responsibility and freedom are central values." Big Food can keep government at bay (partly by calling it "Big Government") by playing to the commonly held core American belief that everyone's success or failure in life is largely up to him or her.

Brownell and Warner sum up Big Food's framing strategy this way:

- Focus on personal responsibility as the cause of the nation's unhealthy diet;
- Raise fears that government action usurps personal freedom;
- Vilify critics with language characterizing them as totalitarians—the food police, leaders of a nanny state, and even "food fascists"—and accuse them of desiring to strip people of their civil liberties;
- Disparage studies critical of the industry as "junk science";
- Emphasize the importance of physical activity over diet;
- State there are no good or bad foods per se; hence no food or food type (soft drinks, fast food, etc.) should be targeted for change;
- Plant doubt when concerns are raised about the industry.

Big Food's sophisticated communication tactics are to be admired. The industry's financial success and phenomenal global reach could not have been achieved without a plan to neutralize public opposition to products that have been proven to cause immense harm. But sometimes you have to take the high road in the communication game by also putting forth a positive message. Take the commencement address delivered at the Georgia Institute of Technology in 2009 by John F. Brock III, the CEO of Coca-Cola: "I am optimistic about the future. . . . Maybe you expect to hear such optimism from a guy who sells a product like Coca-Cola that invites you to 'open happiness.' But consider this theme for a moment. Coca-Cola operates in more corners of the world than any other enterprise. It's been said that after the world 'hello,' Coca-Cola is the most recognized word in the world. Our business has chosen the idea of 'happiness' as the best way to connect our brand with billions of people in more than 200 countries. [This] was a *thoroughly analyzed decision* [my emphasis] about what speaks to the aspirations of people today." Who would have thought that the key to happiness was Coca-Cola!

But sometimes the happy face frowns. More recently, the industrial food system has "gone negative" with a series of attacks and withering critiques leveled against the alternative food system. It may be in response to the onslaught of books (*Omnivore's Dilemma, Fast Food Nation*), films (*Food, Inc.*), and the endless stream of articles that have pummeled the industrial food system over the past three or four years, but clearly David has found his range and is landing enough rocks on Goliath to elicit a loud and angry counterattack.

For some reason "locavores"—those who propose that more of our food should be produced and consumed locally—have been the object of much scorn by the industrial food system. Why people who like to buy tomatoes at farmers' markets or grow a few of their own in the backyard should be singled out for such abuse suggests that Big Food is feeling pressure. Tom Keane in the *Boston Globe* chides locavores for irrational sentimentality: eating local "may get us back in touch with our roots, but it's a ridiculous way to run an economy. . . . For some reason we still cling to the notion that it's better if we have farmers scattered all about" than to have them concentrated in certain parts of the country. Steve Dubner joined the chorus with an opinion piece in the *New York Times* titled "Do We Really Need a Few Billion Locavores?" He attacked the local food movement from the economic side, claiming that it's not cheaper to grow your own food and that it's not necessarily better for the environment either. George Will took on those who turn their nose up at McDonald's in his *Washington Post* column, calling them "food fascists [who] purse their lips and wax censorious at the mere mention of McDonald's." My God, I'd better douse my veg-etable garden with gasoline, light a match to it, and start eating more Big Macs before I become responsible for mass starvation.

These are only a few examples of how the media has been put in service on behalf of the industrial food system. By supposedly de-bunking some of the myths of the alternative food system, or find-ing some of the chinks in its armor, they are heeding the advice of all good football coaches: "The best defense is a good offense." If it can soften up the opposition with a good cannon shelling, then the industrial food system can pave the way for its final assault on the holdouts.

GOING GLOBAL

And like companies from all industrial sectors throughout modern history, America's food sector can always find someplace in the world where it will get a little less heat. The *New York Times* did an extensive exposé on Smithfield Foods' development of new hog production facilities overseas, including in Mexico, Poland, and Romania, and processing facilities in Britain, France, Spain, and China. As the U.S.'s largest hog processor and one of the largest processors of beef and turkey, the corporation had over $11 billion in sales in 2008. Smithfield fine-tuned its system of hog production in the early 1990s in North Carolina: "With assembly-line effi-ciency, sows churn out litters three or four times a year. Within 300 days, a 270-pound pig is ready for slaughter." But mountains of waste, polluted waterways, dead wildlife, fouled air, and ongoing labor strife have earned the company a permanent place in the pan-theon of corporate villainy. While no one is suggesting that Smith-field is leaving the U.S. anytime soon, they now have 550 employees in Poland, where they have produced over 1 million hogs, 850 em-ployees in Romania, where they have produced 580,000 hogs, and 2,500 employees in Mexico, where they have produced 467,000 hogs. Yes, it's the same old story—find a place that's hungry for economic development and not too persnickety about environmental regulations, and that has a cheap and compliant labor force, and your profit margins will zoom. But as you're driving out the small, local producers who have been the backbone of these countries' food systems for centuries, you're also spreading a kind of industrial food system hegemony across the globe.

In an attempt to catch up to the near-universal name recognition of Coca-Cola and McDonald's, Burger King has been conducting "taste comparisons" with Hmong people in Thailand, Inuits in Greenland, and villagers in Romania. Derrick Jackson of the *Boston Globe* labeled the practice a modern form of colonization and compared it to the colonial white settlers in Massachusetts spreading disease to the area's Native Americans. "The Westernization of the global diet, led by America's fast food giants, is helping spread obesity and diabetes as it has never been seen before." Like Big Tobacco did with developing countries to which it exported cigarettes, Big Food is now "exporting" obesity and diabetes to places like Guatemala, the Republic of the Congo, and Bangladesh, where diabetes rates are expected to triple. A doubling to near tripling of diabetes rates is expected as well in China, Mexico, India, and Brazil. The U.S. may not make clothing, shoes, or wide-screen TVs anymore, but we sure know how to make a damn good hamburger. More importantly, we are using the great American marketing machine to permanently brand consumers far and wide with our fast food products. Once they're hooked, once they're indoctrinated in the ways of American gastronomy, we'll own them.

DEMOCRACY UNDER SIEGE

This brings us to what may be the most egregious power play—the industrial food system's attempts to undermine democracy. Using high-paid lobbyists in Washington and in state capitals, the industrial food system has directed a considerable amount of financial resources to secure favorable regulations, pass new legislation that will prevent opponents from taking action against it, and oppose legislation that it regards as counter to its interests. In the case of seed giant Monsanto, a host of intimidating tactics has been used against farmers who have been accused of collecting the seed from their GMO crops, a violation of the company's licensing agreement that a buyer must purchase new seed each year. Farmers have been followed by Monsanto's agents, pictures have been taken of the farmers to prove that big corporate brother is watching, and lawsuits have been filed, sometimes resulting in substantial fines.

Holding aside the arguments for and against GMO seed for a moment, it is interesting how corporations get their way and can change our lives without debate, without our formal consent; and on those occasions when we do object openly, they use every means possible to override public concerns. In an excellent piece of reporting, Donald Barlett and James Steele documented Monsanto's abuses of corporate power in *Vanity Fair,* including its reliance on "a shadowy army of private agents in the American heartland to strike fear into farm country." One Monsanto nonseed product that has provoked outrage is Posilac, the company's branded artificial bovine growth hormone (rBGH), which increases the cow's natural production of milk. In an effort to clear the field of those who do not subscribe to its religion, Monsanto has filed claims with the Federal Trade Commission against dairy products that advertise their milk as "rBGH free." Whether artificial hormones in milk are dangerous to humans or cows isn't the question; Monsanto is claiming you can't say your product doesn't use them!

In Pennsylvania, according to Barlett and Steele, Monsanto prevailed upon the state's agriculture secretary, Dennis Wolff, to prohibit dairies from labeling their milk as produced without the use of artificial hormones. Agreeing with the industry, Wolff said that such a label implies that milk produced with rBGH is not safe, an odd argument to make, since such products with the USDA organic certification logo don't imply that nonorganic products are not safe because they are produced without artificial chemicals, etc. The secretary's action provoked a firestorm of opposition that forced Pennsylvania's governor Edward Rendell to overturn the decision, saying, "The public has a right to complete information about how the milk they buy is produced."

In Hawaii, which is one of the nation's leading producers of GMO seed, numerous bills were filed in the state's 2009 legislative session to protect consumers and farmers against GMO products. Of course, Big Food organized against these bills, many of which were nothing more than "right to know" bills.

Another bill filed the same year in the Montana legislature sought to protect farmers from on-farm searches conducted by Monsanto when in hot pursuit of an alleged seed violator. The bill merely extended the same right that a homeowner enjoys under the U.S. Constitution to be free from unwarranted search and seizure to private sector investigations. The Montana Seed Trade Association, the Beet Growers Association of Montana, and the Montana Farm Bureau Federation all testified, predictably, against the bill. Representatives from Monsanto itself didn't show up at the public hearing. No need to. The corporation had given a private presentation to members of the legislative committee that had cognizance over the bill just a week prior at the Montana Club. As of this writing, biotechnology seed companies and state-based industrial food system interests have successfully blocked all state legislation to protect the rights of all non-GMO-seed users and property owners adjoining GMO-using farms.

In a case that will be discussed in more detail later, Boulder County (Colorado) held a series of hearings to decide whether to allow the use of GMO sugar beet seeds on county-owned farmland. The main claim by the farmers requesting the use of that seed was that there was no other (non-GMO) seed available in the marketplace. Will that be how the final decision is made when we are asked to choose between food products? Will the industrial food system respond, "We've taken them all away, except one, which happens to be the one we make—whether you like it or not. The choice, therefore, is between eating and not eating."

PART II
LEADING THE CHARGE

Whatever makes life vivid and delightful is the heavenly bread. . . . In sowing the seed man has his contact with earth, with sun and rain: and he must not break the contact. . . . And man must not lose this supreme state of consciousness . . . or he has lost the best part of him.

—D.H. LAWRENCE

How will the millions of alternative food adherents become billions? Will the alternative food system just hold its ground, perhaps making marginal gains over time, or might it one day triumph over the industrial food system? Is it possible that a new order might emerge, founded on the principles of democracy, intimacy, and mass participation in our food system? Or will the Grand Inquisitor's prediction come true: that the great mass of people will succumb to "miracle, mystery, and authority" in return for the certainty of bread?

To send the Grand Inquisitor packing will take more than a multitude of smaller-scale local food projects and a commitment by the industrial food system to modify some of its practices. Yes, those can be regarded as helpful steps in a set of partial reforms, but the net result will remain the same: the more we place our confidence in others rather than in ourselves, the more things will remain the same. As the song by the Who says, "Meet the new boss; same as the old boss." The greatest risk we face by giving away our participation in the food system is not only the loss of healthy food and a clean environment; it is the atrophy of basic human skills necessary to preserving not only our lives, but also our souls.

What follows in part II are nine chapters that provide a host of actual examples from around the United States (and one from South Korea). They illustrate the kind of approaches that, if adopted widely, would be capable of fomenting a wholesale change in attitudes toward our food system. Furthermore, if these approaches could be multiplied, they might very well be capable, within two generations, of making the alternative food system (may we also call it the good food system?) the dominant one by 2050. We might actually dethrone the Grand Inquisitor.

The approaches fall into three categories: food production (chapters 4–6), food education (chapters 7–9), and food democracy (chapters 10–12). In various ways all three deal with fundamental problems—I'll call them innate fears—that we as human beings and society have evolved since World War II. We fear putting our hands in the soil and resist the idea that we should get hot and sweaty participating in even limited efforts to produce our own food. We fear cooking our food, hesitating to employ unprocessed ingredients to assemble simple but tasty dishes. And we fear raising our own voice in public policy arenas in pursuit of the values that we hold dear. All three fears are often transmitted from one generation to the next, with the result that fewer of us grow some quantity of our food, prepare meals from whole food, or participate in public forums that are designed to change food policy. All three fears alienate us from our food system, and the wider the gap between us and our food, the more opportunity there is for the industrial food system to exploit our fears and drive us further into its camp.

To build alternatives and assert our independence requires that we rebuild our confidence as both individuals and communities. In effect, the dominance of the industrial food system is related as much to a crisis of confidence in ourselves as it is to that system's ability to use its amassed power to control policy makers, markets, and consumers. Since a frontal assault on that power would be as futile as it would be foolish, the path to victory is by way of a renaissance in food knowledge and a reemergence of citizen democracy. The following chapters tell the story of some who have trodden that path.

CHAPTER 4
MAURICE SMALL
AND THE GREENING OF CLEVELAND

Maurice Small walked into the hotel lobby where I sat one chilly morning barely two days into spring. I had met him once briefly, and had seen him in a locally produced documentary film about food and farming in northeast Ohio. But these glimpses hadn't prepared me for the tall, lanky black man who ambled through the revolving doors. Smiling and bespectacled, he sported a mass of salt-and-pepper Rasta curls that gushed like a fountain from a multihued headband.

We hopped into his 1974 pickup. Like its owner, the truck was a working vehicle—not beautiful but ready to do whatever had to be done. Seeing me struggle with my coffee container, Maurice apologized for the truck's lack of cup holders, but he was decidedly unapologetic about the cab's disheveled appearance or the malfunctioning passenger seatbelt. Comfort and safety were not the day's priorities. Seeing Cleveland's urban gardens was.

Heading east from a downtown that had seen better times, we were soon in neighborhoods where residential one- and two-family homes mixed randomly with commercial structures and vacant lots. On Euclid Avenue, once a proud golden mile of millionaire mansions, the properties alternated between abandoned houses, barren lots, and dingy small businesses. Like a barroom brawler who has seen too many fights, the neighborhood's smile was missing every other tooth.

It's in places like this where the nonprofit organization City

Fresh has planted its flag. Maurice's employer, it is the group that is organizing a wide range of food production and distribution options across the northeast Ohio region. The organization is cultivating commercial growers as well as urban gardeners while developing outlets for their crops at the same time. Besides tapping into the purchasing power of large institutions such as hospitals and colleges to create markets for these producers, it has also developed what are called "Fresh Stops" in low- and moderate-income Cleveland neighborhoods. Operating much like a community-supported agriculture farm, Fresh Stops are sites that distribute locally produced food in communities that are particularly lacking in any high-quality, affordable food stores. At the growing end of the spectrum, City Fresh provides gardening training and marketing assistance for the urban market. On the consumer side, nutrition education is provided to help households learn how to shop for and prepare fresh, local food.

By partnering with a number of groups, including Oberlin College's New Agrarian Center, the Cleveland Health Department, and the Ohio State University Cooperative Extension, City Fresh has trained fifty-one urban garden entrepreneurs, developed thirteen garden sites, and opened fifteen Fresh Stops. Cleveland, like Detroit, Chicago, Milwaukee, and other cities, grapples with a surfeit of vacant land; City Fresh is trying to convert the city's deficits into assets—or, to put it another way, turn lemons into lemonade.

Maurice steered down Standard Street, a spacious, tree-lined boulevard. But I quickly realized that the airiness of the landscape was simply a result of demolished buildings and empty parking lots. Pointing to a gaping pit in the ground that was nearly a city block long, Maurice told me that it was the site of a former school built in the 1930s (prior to that time the site had been a farm). It had been "deconstructed," meaning that it had been carefully disassembled so that people could make use of the building's wide wooden floorboards, beams, and joists for other building projects. Two or three large piles of bricks, each scrubbed of their graying mortar, lay at the pit's edge. These were being used by many of Cleveland's 4,000 urban gardeners, who were recycling them for garden-bed curbs, walkway pavers, and supports for raised planting units. People were seizing every useable molecule for reuse across the breadth of Cuyahoga County.

"Here's the Standard Garden," said Maurice as we pulled into a large parking lot devoid of motor vehicles and white lines, but nurturing a few blades of spring grass that had muscled their way through the asphalt cracks. Piled against an irregular series of brick walls that form the site's northern boundary was a mound of shredded tree mulch and compost, densely packed and three feet high. This vast heap covered approximately 2,000 square feet of pavement, forming a mini mesa top. Atop this assemblage of biomass several troughs had been dug, backfilled with topsoil, and now were waiting patiently for some warmer weather for seeds and plants.

Even more unusual than the planting medium was the irrigation system. It consisted of one twenty-foot plastic gutter slung off the edge of garage rooftops that adjoined the garden's edge. The six-inch diameter half-pipe caught water from several roofs and channeled it into a series of eight fifty-gallon blue plastic drums, each one connected to the next with a small plastic tube—when one drum filled, the overflow was sent into the next and so on. Since there was no water source on the property, this jury-rigged system, combined with Mother Nature's unpredictable beneficence, was what made the garden grow.

The garden was constructed—a process consisting of moving hundreds of wheelbarrows full of mulch—by community volunteers. Though the immediate neighbors have sanctioned the garden, which confers a kind of legitimacy and protection for the site, it is planted, tended, and harvested by two Cleveland locals known as the Levine sisters, Emmie and Jessica. The produce is sold at farmers' markets, Fresh Stops, and, in a kind of urban twist on the old sharecropping system, is distributed to the garden's neighbors. While no one would equate the latter to protection money, Maurice noted that the parking lot where the garden rests was once a place to leave junk cars, conduct drug deals, and engage in all manner of malfeasance. Now that there's a garden and people who care about it, the bad stuff doesn't happen anymore—at least not there.

Cleveland is a tough place, one that is not likely to achieve posterchild status for its version of new urbanism anytime soon. The crumbling hulls of steel mills and the skeletal remains of rust-belt detritus still remain. Since 1960 the city's population has plunged from nearly 1 million to fewer than 500,000, losing 100,000 people since 2002 alone (a number that is surpassed only by the refugees who fled Katrina-ravaged New Orleans). Even before the Armageddon of the nation's mortgage and housing crisis, Cleveland led the nation in foreclosures: a staggering 10,000 from 2006 to 2008.

Foreclosures and outmigration mean abandoned housing. City officials estimate that between 10,000 and 15,000 homes are vacant; that's almost one in every ten. And abandoned housing is frequently dealt with by demolitions, which then create more empty land. While the actual number of vacant lots is not known, it is fair to assume that Cleveland could easily rival some Iowa farm counties—complete with mega-farms, monster tractors, and air-conditioned combines—if all those lots could be assembled into one contiguous urban parcel.

When mainline industries like steel or auto downsize their operations or leave a place entirely, the biggest employers and most powerful players then become the public and private institutions such as government, universities, and hospitals. They are either too rooted historically in the community or see reasonable market opportunities no matter what the change in demographics. From a cynical perspective, some institutions may even see upside potential in downtrending social and economic indicators.

The venerable Cleveland Medical Clinic, which physically dominates the city's eastern half, continues to expand, perhaps in some inverse proportion to the area's overall decline in health. Though a beacon of prosperity in an otherwise depressed area, the medical complex is surrounded by the kind of food desert common in urban America. The area is bereft of decent grocery stores, but has a relatively high proportion of fast food joints, including the McDonald's franchise that operates *inside the clinic's main lobby*. These are the physical conditions that, when mixed with poverty and poor education, produce a breeding ground for obesity, diabetes, and cardiovascular disease.

Go just a little further east and this recipe for a public health disaster becomes even stronger, as does the opportunity for cynicism. Crossing the border between Cleveland and East Cleveland is not noticeable to the casual observer. But gradually there is a sense that things have gone from bad to worse. We passed a former Tops Supermarket, probably 40,000 square feet with two or three acres of parking, which made it a decent-size store even by suburban standards. It had been closed for four years when the Giant Eagle chain bought it out. According to Maurice, the store was very busy on the first and fifteenth of each month when the community's largely poor and African American population was flush with public assistance cash. It apparently struggled the rest of the time, eventually closing its doors for good. Now, the closest supermarket is almost 4 miles away, which might as well be 100 miles if you don't have a car and must rely on public transit. About the only place that seemed to be thriving, aside from the Taco Bells and Burger Kings, was a locally owned rib joint that has been so successful it has seven locations throughout Cleveland.

Just a few blocks from where fifteen people waited at a bus stop, all of them overweight and most of them obese, sits Huron Hospital, a satellite facility of the Cleveland Clinic. The hospital specializes in the treatment of diabetes and other diet-related illnesses like cardiovascular disease. It serves the community with hundreds of jobs; it often treats people who have no health insurance coverage at all; its cafeteria is modeling such "green" behaviors as the composting of food wastes and changing over to biodegradable utensils and plates. It even gives its waste cooking oil to City Fresh to power the latter's produce-delivery vehicles. To most people, that might sound like a highly responsible public institution, but in Maurice's words, it's also part of "a perfect system—no supermarkets, lots of fast food joints, diabetes running rampant, and a first-class diabetes treatment center just around the corner."

Contradictions like these are lodged in Maurice's consciousness in the same way they are for any aware African American who grew up in late twentieth-century America. For some, however, the pain is too great and anger eventually consumes them. But for those like Maurice, a combination of survival instincts, caring parents, and spiritual faith have enabled them to outmaneuver what might have otherwise been a grim fate. They climb over their despair like embattled troopers mounting a pile of rubble, grabbing pieces of useable masonry along the way with which to build new foundations. In Maurice's case, the trooper is clutching a rake and a hoe instead of an AK-47.

"I got tired seeing the same vacant lots that I've been looking at ever since I was a kid," he proclaimed with only a smidgen of bitterness, the most I'd hear him express in our two days together. We stood on a postage-stamp-size piece of open ground next to one of the Huron's smaller outbuildings staring at Maurice's most recent horticultural creation. It was a twenty-foot by fifty-foot garden shouldered on all four sides by two courses of hay bales. The space in between had been backfilled with several dump-truck loads of compost and earth. The garden, which has been growing vegetables since May 2008, was wedged into a spot that had a high brick wall on one side ("We'll be growing espaliered fruits trees against it," said Maurice) and a small hedge on the other ("That's where the raspberries are going"). In the only remaining unplanted corner was the compost pile, which was now in the process of being filled with biodegradable waste (safe and hygienic) from the hospital.

While admiring the compact image of sustainability that lay

before me as well as the industry of Maurice and his colleagues, I wondered out loud if projects like this were really enough to turn around the kind of social and economic dysfunction that I had just witnessed only blocks away. At that point Maurice grew animated. He lowered his gangly frame to the ground in a basketball crouch as if challenging me to dribble past him. Pointing to the garden, he said, "We're going to make this the model, man! You gotta tweak 'em; get that virus in their [the institution's] veins. Yes, it starts in a poor community because a wealthy community wouldn't accept a compost pile."

It was then that I realized Maurice had a plan. He wasn't just some hip-hop version of Johnny Appleseed planting vacant lots across Cuyahoga County. Gardens like the one he was now jumping up and down in were part of a longer-term, hands-on vision of revival that used the resources of empty land, institutional strength (including a dash of white guilt), and small groups of willing neighbors and sheepish teenagers to make something happen now. In his opinion, this would take people down the path to bigger, more difficult tasks like building housing and creating good-paying jobs. "I'm crazy, man. I'm not patient. People are dying all over these communities," he howled as if in pain. "I can't wait for the politicians or policy to turn this around. This [the garden] is the kind of practical politics I'm talking about."

Another one of Cleveland's institutional assets is Case Western Reserve University, renowned as "the MIT of the Midwest," which sits proudly at the city's eastern edge. Its nearly 10,000 students and 2,600 faculty are known to frequently eat three meals a day (even techies need food). Maurice and his partners at City Fresh, along with hundreds of city gardeners and dozens of area farmers, saw the opportunity to grow and sell food to this formidably large institution of higher learning. As a systems kind of guy, Maurice was as enamored with the output potential—compostable waste—as he was with the input potential of locally produced fruits and vegetables. The deal was made even richer when they joined forces with Oberlin College, a small, ultraliberal academic citadel only fifty miles from Cleveland, and only too happy to partner in a project with so much environmental and social upside potential.

Today, through a combination of the area's farmers and city gardeners (who are also sometimes called farmers), $2 million a year of locally produced food is finding its way into the stomachs of college professors and the future engineers of America. In contrast to the tall, bushy-haired, African American Maurice, Joe Gentile, one of Case Western's food service managers, is short, bald, and Italian. But their shared love of good food and the easy rapport they've established through their business relationship transcends all outward differences. (Paying Joe the highest compliment, Maurice confided to me later, "I love Italians; they're so passionate about food.")

Maurice proudly showed me the food displayed throughout the cafeteria line and dining hall. "Those are City Fresh onions; the apples over there are from one of our local apple orchards; the beef they serve is locally produced." This being late March in Ohio, the variety of local food items was impressive. Maurice noted that cauliflower, cabbage, and potatoes, held in cold storage, were also being sold this late in the year to Oberlin and Case as part of City Fresh's weekly deliveries. Starting with the 2009 growing season, City Fresh extended their delivery period from August to June.

City Fresh is lucky in one sense: both Case Western and Oberlin's dining services are managed by Bon Appetite, perhaps the nation's most progressive food service company. A walk through this particular cafeteria unit at Case is like a walk through the Modern Food Gallery of the Politically Correct. The walls are adorned with uniformly designed, high-production graphics of every imaginable label certifying the humaneness, organicness, and downright righteousness of nearly every product that will pass your lips during your tenure in these hallowed halls. The daily menu, nailed to the foyer's wall with the same assertiveness with which Martin Luther affixed his ninety-five theses to the doors of the Wittenberg Cathedral, announces in bold print the farm from which each dish's ingredients originated. And in an effort to reduce waste, Joe Gentile has placed a big chart next to the disposal station tracking the weekly reduction in uneaten food.

But Bon Appetite's sense of responsibility is not limited to what is served at each of its 400 dining units nationwide. In 2009 it waded into the murky waters of fairness and justice as they affect farm workers in the heart of the South's tomato-growing region, Immokalee, Florida. Responding to a plethora of labor abuses—low wages, substandard working conditions, and even convictions for slavery—Bon Appetite is using its purchasing muscle (the threat to buy its 5 million pounds of tomatoes elsewhere) to compel growers to increase pay and improve working conditions. Such actions are indeed bold and take the pursuit of fairness and justice to new levels, particularly as it sometimes requires a higher level of commitment and business risk to buy from a motley assortment of local growers whose farms range in size from hundreds of acres to 2,000 square feet. Seasonality, unpredictability of supply, and unevenness in quality are the realities of patronizing small, local agriculture that could easily pluck the remaining hairs from Joe Gentile's scalp. In spite of these obstacles, Bon Appetite is doing well, and with the assistance of aggregators like City Fresh, building the wealth of Cleveland and its surrounding region.

As with the "viral" effect that Maurice hopes for from his community gardens, he sees the food connection to institutions like Case as the battering ram that might break down the walls between town and gown. It takes no more than a couple of right turns out of the pristine, tree-lined Case campus to enter a very different world. No liberal sensibilities are required to see the line that separates privilege and wealth from the struggle of Glenville, the all-black, lower-income neighborhood that abuts the Case campus. Abandoned housing mixed with renovations in progress and empty lots in all manner of disarray (except those that Maurice has targeted for community gardens) immediately alter the perspective of someone who just enjoyed the respite from urban grit granted by the Case oasis.

Without intending to provoke Maurice, I asked him what he thought of the contrast. His demeanor, usually mellow, immediately turned passionate. He said that Case students never cross that all-too-evident line. "White people left this neighborhood thirty years ago, and there's no dialogue between the community and the university. And as far as I can tell, the community doesn't want to talk to the university because they don't trust them."

Once the smoke had cleared, Maurice's innate sense of optimism returned, as did his tenacious grip on hope. "I believe that we can get the [university's] chefs to come to the neighborhood and work with the gardeners and families. There's hope that people in the neighborhood can sell to the university, even if it's only $20 of lettuce, because you know what, that $20 might be the first paycheck some people from this community ever got." A new working bond between the university and the surrounding neighborhoods is not just a one-way street as far as Maurice is concerned. "The students will benefit from actually experiencing this place. Right now, they don't know a thing about it even though they live only a few blocks away. Food and gardening can be the way to start the dialogue."

Later, over lunch, I asked Maurice how he would describe himself—community organizer, servant leader, or just plain old agitator. He was quiet for a few moments as he mulled over the options. "I'm a hustler," he decided with a wry smile. "I move between different communities and build bridges so that they can share with each other." Unlike a swaggering *Super Fly* version, the hustler image that Maurice conjured up reminded me of a bee, as in Mohammed Ali's "Float like a butterfly, sting like a bee," or more literally the necessary insect that moves with easy grace from flower to flower. "Like a chameleon, I'll become whatever the people need me to be," he went on to explain. "I have to hustle to start five gardens and help with three diabetes programs. A farmer has 2,200 pounds of green beans that he harvested but has no place to sell them. I have to hustle up a market. I have to hustle for a child who can't read the back of a seed packet, or for the ladies who run an after-school program but who are about to give up because they have no funding."

In Cleveland's Tremont neighborhood, another side of Maurice's hustling style was revealed. The community is on the city's west side and has a comfortable mixed-income, shady suburban feel to it. With a large park at its center and located not far from the city's Westside Public Market, Tremont has achieved a kind of social and economic stability built, in part, around food, especially gardens and restaurants. In one area that is only a short distance from the old steel mills, there are twelve good restaurants, including Lolita's, owned by Michael Simon, aka television's Iron Chef, now a genuine local superhero.

According to Maurice, chef Simon is also a great guy, whose celebrity has not inflated his ego or made him difficult to work with. On the contrary, Simon has been leading the charge in buying food from local farmers and gardeners. With the help of Maurice and a team of local kids, six raised beds were installed in Lolita's tiny backyard (raised beds are generally required in this area because the mills polluted the underlying soil beyond redemption). Most of the vegetables and herbs find their way into the restaurant's kitchen, but the garden serves another purpose as well; when children from a nearby elementary school come by to tend it, they also cultivate their emerging interests in plants, worms, and soil. And chef Simon carries the sustainability ball even further downfield by composting his waste and pumping his spent cooking oil into City Fresh's delivery vans.

Brokering these kinds of win-win relationships are Maurice's forte. Using the assets of the place, whatever they are and from wherever they come, has created a nearly endless web of opportunities that lead to more gardens, more farmers' markets, more kids getting their hands into dirt, more worms turning more food waste into more compost, and more local food for everybody. His is an expansive vision that assembles a series of steps from the raw materials at hand into an ever-ascending staircase that takes all those who want to climb it to a higher and better place.

The waitress set our meals before us. Since Maurice is a vegetarian, his dish presented a colorful array of vegetables set enticingly on a bed of pasta. He looked reverently down at the dish for a moment, and then did something I've never seen anyone do before: pulling out his phone camera and holding it twelve inches above his plate, he snapped a shot of the food. Maurice is a Seventh-Day Adventist, and for a moment I thought I was witnessing some religious practice heretofore unknown to me. Seeing the quizzical look on my face, he held the camera screen up to me and scrolled backward through a series of photos, all depicting previous meals—a veritable photo gallery of breakfasts, lunches, and dinners consumed by Maurice over the past week. "I look back on the photos," he explained, "to remind me of where the meal came from, what restaurant I may have eaten it in, who prepared it, and how it smelled and tasted." Not only did he feel that this was a way to honor his food and all who contributed to it—from the worms that enriched the soil to the person who placed the completed dish before him—it was a way to create an authentic bond between him and nature: a oneness that is as molecular as it is spiritual.

For Maurice this concept of authenticity is central to who he is and extends as well to his relationship with his community. When he feels a sense of authenticity flowing through his veins and in the world around him, he feels empowered. As he works with others to grow food, and through that process builds strong bridges to upscale restaurants and powerful institutions, not only does he create a more unified and practical approach to community development, he is enabling others to discover their own latent powers.

"The secret fortune is joy in our hands. Welcome evermore to gods and men is the self-helping man. For him all doors are flung wide," wrote Emerson in his essay "Self-Reliance." Maurice acknowledges the oppression and poverty of the people. He knows racism the way that any black man does. But rather than languish in some sense of perpetual victimhood, Maurice embraces all around him—black and white, poor and rich, young and old—as "associates" who have hands, time, and a God-given power to release untapped energies that will lift their souls, build their communities, and fling doors wide open.

CHAPTER 5
ME AND MY MEAT

Have you ever gone into a crowded, filthy restaurant where the flies are circling the food, the floor is littered with the spillage of previous diners, and the odor of decay assaults your olfactory sense? The sight and smell of such a place are usually accompanied by the sound of patrons emitting an unappetizing chorus of smacking, slurping, and snuffling noises. Unless starvation is imminent, you'll probably escape this culinary hell before the surly waitress has thrown the yellow-stained plastic menu at you.

Now imagine that the food you eat comes from animals that are raised on factory farms where a similar "ambiance" prevails—chickens confined to cages just a couple of feet square, flies swarming over cows that are standing snout-to-tail in muck up to their knees, and hogs treading concrete floors in buildings that deny them both daylight and the thing that makes hogs happiest, rooting about in God's good earth.

THE BAD AND THE UGLY
Take a drive through Don Opplinger's Land and Cattle Feedlot in Clovis, New Mexico, and you'll see 35,000 head of beef cattle confined in pens that march across the flat, treeless terrain. The constant shuffling of hooves raises a bacteria-laden dust cloud that's carried by the prevailing winds across Clovis into west Texas, where it joins the plumes emanating from hundreds of other beef and dairy yards. At one end of the Clovis complex sits a giant lagoon

that catches all manner of farm effluvia, including wastewater, chemicals, urine, and antibiotics.

My pickup truck tour of the penned areas was led by a veteran local farmer who told me to roll up the windows to keep the flies and the worst of the stench out. I was surprised that someone who had spent sixty-five years around livestock and assorted farm operations wasn't entirely immune to this environment. We had gained entry to an area of the feedlot that was off-limits to the general public purely on the basis of the smiles and winks he gave the farm's sole office worker, a bored-looking middle-aged woman who was the only person "guarding" the facility. During the few minutes I spent in the feedlot's office as my guide chatted her up, I noticed nearly a dozen scented candles strewn about the place. I asked her what they were for, expecting the answer I got: "Sometimes this place stinks so bad, I have to light them to cover up the smell."

In the narrow strip of land that separates the fenced pens from the farm's main dirt road lay the carcasses of dead cows ("downers," in the parlance of the cattle industry), their eyes bugged out, tongues dangling obscenely, and bellies swollen in the ninety-degree heat.

The tallest structure in the complex is a feed mill that steams and rolls corn into a flake, the feedlot's biggest input that will take a 450-pound calf to a market-size 1,250-pound steer in eight months. The calves come from all over America for fattening at Opplinger's. When they're ready for market, they are shipped to slaughter and packing plants owned by Cargill or Tyson in Freeona or Plainview, Texas, where they are killed at the rate of 5,000 per day. Depending on the price at the auction house, Mr. Opplinger is likely to receive $85 per hundredweight, or about $1,100 per cow, just a few pennies per pound above his break-even point. But lest you shed a tear for Mr. Opplinger, you should know that he and the other farm operations he owns in Nebraska and Texas collectively received $1,522,037 in USDA benefits between 2003 and 2005, which placed him among the top five recipients of commodity certificate benefits in the United States during that period, according to the *Washington Post*. Yes, our taxes support this operation and others like it, referred to as "concentrated animal feeding operations," or CAFOs, by government agencies.

Call it what you want, but a feedlot will never be Old McDonald's Farm. When it rains hard, the cattle are up to their knees in mud. When it's dry, dust is everywhere, and the flies, well, they are as thick as flies. But if you eat beef, and most Americans do, chances are pretty good it comes from a feedlot like this. They are capital-intensive operations—Opplinger's has at least $20 million worth of cattle housed in a $10-million yard—that produce beef with nearly factory-like precision. For instance, it used to be that you brought the cow to the feed—namely, pasture and grass—but today the opposite is true. Using a system of railroads and grain elevators—all of which have their own legacy of public subsidy—that delivers cheap grain (also subsidized) from the Midwest, feedlot operators can have a fattened steer ready for market in no time. This is why beef, in some form or another, is an affordable item in almost everyone's shopping cart.

I eat meat because I have yet to find much in life that competes with a tender rib eye accompanied by a good bottle of zinfandel. But the explosion of factory livestock farms is not about one's choice to eat the flesh of other species. It is about what CAFOs are doing to our water, air, land, the social and economic fabric of rural communities, the health of their residents, and yes, those animals that end up on our plates.

Most of us enjoy meat without the fuss and muss of raising livestock or living near a factory farm that does. And we do so quite cheaply. In fact, U.S. shoppers spend less on food as a percentage of their total annual household expenditures than the people of any other country in the world. But this is because factory farms and other industrial-scale food producers don't pay for the natural resources they have squandered and defiled, the farm labor they have exploited, the declining health of residents who live near their operations, or the animals they have used far beyond their biological capabilities.

But if you're looking for the pinnacle of meat madness, look no further than factory hog farms. The odor they generate is so intense it would knock a buzzard off a shit-wagon. In a building 100 feet long and just 9 feet high, as many as 20,000 hogs are confined their entire lives. After five months, the mature hogs are sent off to the slaughterhouse to have their throats slit and carcasses dipped in chemical vats to loosen their skins. No doubt for these sentient beings their death, gruesome though it is, is a welcome relief from the life that preceded it. According to Anita Poole, legal counsel for the Kerr Center, an Oklahoma organization that has fought that state's hog industry, "The average Joe Blow who might stumble into a hog facility would never want to eat pork again."

Texas County is in Oklahoma's Panhandle region. In 1990 it had 11,000 hogs, but today, according to the Kerr Center, the number has swollen to well over 1 million. For a region that was in economic decline, the offer by Seaboard Farms to locate an industrial-style hog operation was too good to resist. It would reinvigorate the flagging economy, create desperately needed jobs, and refill the empty school desks. But there was a cost. Seaboard demanded and received approximately $60 million in local and state government assistance (if these were poor people asking for help, it would be called welfare). This worked out to $27,552 per new job, which in the slightly screwy calculus of local economic development might not be too bad if the jobs paid $20 per hour, but the average Seaboard wage was less than $8. Even in spite of the low wages, the deal might have been justified if the community received a commensurate growth in tax revenues. But by the time the deal was cut, the county received a grand total of $9,700 in taxes each year for the site on which a $100-million business stands.

Factory hog operations not only pay a slim return on the community's investment, they also extract a high price from the surrounding region. Increasingly, factory farm workers in the West and Midwest are Mexican immigrants, and only about half, according to some estimates, are legally documented. They bring with them a host of issues—from the need for English-as-a-second-language school programs to uninsured medical expenses to greater involvement in crime—that these rural communities are unused to and cannot afford. From 1990 to 1997, for instance, crime in Texas County grew by 74 percent, compared to a decline of 12 percent in other rural Oklahoma counties.

The worst problems, however, come from the ungodly amount of manure that this many hogs produce, estimated at about 15 million pounds per day in Texas County. Because of water runoff from factory farms, both groundwater and surface water quality have declined. Even worse, the Ogallala Aquifer upon which the region depends for its water is being depleted at a rapid rate. The Oklahoma Water Resource Board reported that water levels in many Texas County wells had dropped 50 to 100 feet over the last thirty years, due in large part to high water demand created by factory hog operations and the irrigated farm land that supports them.

The same government and private industry partnership that brought CAFOs to America's marginalized rural communities is unable to provide adequate monitoring and regulatory control. Through lax environmental regulations and/or by underfunding the state agencies charged with regulating CAFOs, state governments have used a series of nods, winks, and handshakes to foster CAFO-friendly conditions while at the same time hoodwinking the public into thinking they are protecting its interests. To further guard their flank, factory farm interests have worked aggressively in state legislatures to restrict the ability of local government entities to keep CAFOs out of their communities. And just to be sure, agri-industrial interests consider it an act of "civic duty" for their farmer members to "serve" on local commissions and boards where they prevent local jurisdictions from taking prudent measures to protect the public health.

The hallowed halls of academe have been compromised as well

by CAFO industry "donations" to universities. Rather than use their scientific talents to assess the impact of CAFOs on workers and citizens, research faculty members are required to solve the industry's problems (e.g., disposing of Himalayan mountains of manure). New Mexico State University's research on dairy CAFOs, for instance, was crushed by the dairy industry when a faculty member found evidence of public health threats associated with large dairies. The Kerr Center's Poole said, "Oklahoma State University won't do community impact research because of all the money they get from the pork industry."

Barely 5 percent of U.S. farms now raise 54 percent of the country's beef and dairy cattle. Corporations now produce 98 percent of all poultry. Small to midsize family livestock farms have been going the way of the dinosaur. While "local food movements" and an interest in grass-fed and free-range animal production are gaining traction, it is hard to imagine that it could ever fully substitute for the "blood-dimmed tide" of industrial livestock agriculture at its current rate of growth. Like the factory farmed hog that can only hope for a swift end to his misery, we too might look forward to nothing better than a painful denouement to a system of food production that is by all accounts unsustainable.

Of this we are certain: the water will run out, the land will no longer absorb the torrent of nutrient waste spread upon it, and the overbred, antibiotic- and hormone-injected animals will eventually succumb to their natural limitations and simply give up the ghost. As Anita Poole said, "The factory system of food production will simply implode." And until the citizens of the heartland rise up in sufficient numbers to hold their governments and the corporations that manage CAFOs accountable, there is nothing better to hope for.

THE GOOD

A four-wheel drive tour of the 18,000-acre Ranney Ranch, just east of Corona, New Mexico, is both an exercise in endurance and a reminder that it takes tough work to make a tender steak. At well under 110 pounds, Nancy Ranney, one of several family business partners who own this sweet piece of mesa country, is hardly the image of the hard-riding cowboy you'd normally associate with this rugged landscape. Nevertheless, she steered her pickup truck with gusto and grace over "roads" so rough that they would give pack mules bunions.

Knuckles turning white, perspiration beading my brow, graceful was the last thing I was feeling as the truck crawled over boulders the size of medicine balls. Nancy took her eyes off the road a little longer than I'd have preferred to tell me that her father bought the ranch in 1968 and ran it as a traditional cow-calf operation. "I'd ride my horse all over this ranch, which doesn't seem so big when you're on horseback." I thought that was a funny thing to say about a single property that was bigger than my former home of Hartford, Connecticut.

I was grateful when the turbulence subsided and we headed down a benign stretch of dirt road that took us to the first of a series of metal gates. I poured my rattled frame out of the cab and fumbled with the gate's latch, letting us into a beautiful valley that echoed with the distant lowing of cows. Soon the occasional Black Angus and her week-old calf appeared, pausing from their grazing and nursing to stare back at us. Within a matter of minutes Nancy was deftly maneuvering her way through a sea of black cows whose collective mooing soon drowned out our conversation.

As we passed through another gate, I realized we had just completed the hardest and most stressful part of the ranching experience, namely, getting to the cows. For about twenty-five days on one 700-acre fenced section of pasture, these heifers will contentedly graze while their calves nurse and gradually increase their consumption of grass. At the end of this period, Nancy's ranch manager of twenty-five years, Melvin Johnson, will simply open the gate, allowing the cows to saunter to the next pasture, where time and rest have given its grasses time to rejuvenate.

For the past two years, the Ranney Ranch has been practicing a method of pasture management called rotational grazing. Developed by grass guru Allan Nation and reported on regularly in the *Grassman Stock Farmer,* rotational grazing was once described to me by a New Mexico rancher as the "hardest easiest thing I've ever learned to do." By learning how many cows can be grazed on a certain number of acres for what length of time, ranchers can bring their cattle to market size without purchasing expensive inputs like feed and fertilizer that must be shipped from great distances. The results: more productive and sustainable pastures, healthier animals (ruminants were not "built" to eat grain), cleaner water and air, and a more abundant habitat able to support more species of wildlife.

But as cows are shifted from pasture to pasture, occasionally something goes awry. Nancy and I happened upon one little calf that was caught on the wrong side of the fence and unable to rejoin the herd. We jury-rigged an opening through the wire and I proceeded to chase the poor fellow up and down the fence line hoping he'd eventually find the hole. Probably more frightened by this arm-flapping, dust-churning human than anything he'd seen in his young life, he finally managed to get his wobbly body through our makeshift gate and scampered off in search of his mother. When I told Nancy what fun I'd had, she responded with a smile, "Maybe that will be the cow you eat this year."

For many of these calves, their sojourn in paradise comes to an end about six months later. Starting in late summer, having reached upwards of 700 pounds each on nothing but mother's milk, grass, and water, Nancy's cows are taken two or three at a time to Fort Sumner (New Mexico) Processing, where they will be turned into steaks, roasts, and hamburger. A couple of weeks later, eager customers will show up in their Dodge trucks and Subaru Outbacks to pick up their frozen beef, which has been cut and sized to order. It will then be transported and redistributed to friends and neighbors back across northern New Mexico. And before the outdoor grilling season is over, one of the best rib eyes you'll ever eat will be tempting your palate.

To some, this way of acquiring beef sounds more complicated than picking up a one-pound steak in a plastic-wrapped Styrofoam tray at the supermarket. But consider the alternative. A locally raised New Mexico calf will go to a feedlot in Texas (of the 1.6 million head of cattle that are raised in New Mexico each year, only 63,000 are actually slaughtered there), where it is fed a steady diet of grain shipped in from the Midwest. When that cow has reached market size, it will be shipped from Texas to Kansas or Iowa to processors like Tyson and Cargill which, with a couple of other corporate food giants, control 80 percent of the meat processing in this country. Before those steaks, hamburgers, and roasts reach a retail display case back in New Mexico, they will be shipped to distributors and warehouses in Denver, Colorado. By the time you're standing in the checkout line to pay for your beef, it has traveled 3,000 miles. The meat that Nancy's customers pick up at the slaughter facility in the little town of Fort Sumner will travel only 300 miles. And there's one benefit to this local food chain: every dollar that was spent by the consumer for that beef stayed in New Mexico and supported New Mexico jobs. That slaughter facility employs ten people (a large employer in rural America) and can process only four cows a day.

"Mother's milk and my grass, that's all my cows eat," Nancy fiercely proclaimed. "I don't import feed or energy. I utilize what I have—land, sun, and water—to grow grass." And her relationship with her customers is just as important as the one she has with her animals. With mild chagrin she confessed, "My father sold his cows to a feedlot and I don't know where they went, probably McDonald's, for all I know. I want to know the people who are buying my animals."

And millions of consumers also want to know who raised their animals. In fact, when they take a deep breath and steel themselves, a growing number of eaters are now prepared to face the fact that meat actually comes from animals. These are people who are looking for food with "attributes," which in the case of meat means that they want to know where and how it was raised. They are asking whether the meat is organic, free of hormones and antibiotics, and whether the animal was cared for in a humane way.

Researchers in the fields of nutrition, diet, and animals are demonstrating that these are no longer the idle concerns of an overly sensitive class of food faddists. *Greener Pastures—How Grass-Fed Beef and Milk Contribute to Healthy Eating,* a report prepared by the Union of Concerned Scientists, presented a compilation of twenty-five studies from across the world that compared the nutritional value of grass-fed livestock food products to grain-fed. While modest in its conclusions (there is not yet enough evidence to support all of the health claims made by grass-fed advocates) the report does state that grass-fed beef is lower in total fat than grain-fed, higher in ALA (alpha-linolenic acid), and has a lower omega-6/omega-3 ratio, all of which reduce the risk of coronary heart disease and the incidence of fatal heart attacks. A lower ratio of omega 6/omega 3 fatty acids also promotes higher bone density.

As with many other food products that are supposedly good for you, consumers will wonder if they can afford grass-fed beef. My wife, brother-in-law, and I went in together on one of Nancy's full cows (according to the invoice "a black, white-faced angus," though there was no indication it was the one I had corralled) that weighed in at 655 pounds at the time of slaughter. We paid her $1.95 per pound and then paid Fort Sumner Processing $243 for what came out to 200 pounds of meat. (In spite of my wife's wincing, I also took the tongue, liver, and soup bones, but decided against the hide after conceding that my tanning skills were a little rusty.) After deducting the weight of the bones (I will make stock) and one or two small pieces of meat that I've so far failed to identify, I figured that I was paying about $8 per pound.

When I compared that cost to the various prices for hamburger, roasts, and steaks, which ranged from $3 to $9 per pound at the Albertson's Supermarket, I estimated that my own cow was on average $1 to $2 per pound more than comparable cuts of supermarket beef. Even accounting for my built-in bias, I still think I got a good deal. The meat tastes better (all our dinner guests have agreed), it used far less energy to reach my plate, it never harmed the environment, and 100 percent of my food dollar went to a local rancher and processor.

In a primitive kind of way, I must confess to experiencing a masculine satisfaction from my introduction to grass-fed beef. I was tending one of my Ranney Ranch steaks at the outdoor barbeque—watching the flames lick the meat, the smoke billowing skyward, nostrils filled with the incomparable scent of grilled beef, cold beer in hand. I reflected back on the rough ride across the boulder-strewn ranchland and the "roundup" of my first calf. This had given me a more nuanced sense of the whole food picture, at least the part that includes animals. I sure knew where this portion of my diet came from—I'd experienced that intimately. I had seen a sustainable balance between plants, animals, and water. I had connected other dots such as those related to slaughter, processing, jobs, and economics. Since my beef purchase included some previously unfamiliar cuts, I've been learning how to prepare a wider variety of dishes, including ones that use beef only as a modest complement to a larger selection of plants and grains. Experiencing again a phenomenon I first encountered thirty years ago when I switched from Budweiser to local microbrewed beers, I find I consume less when the quality is higher. One grass-fed hamburger, for instance, satisfies me as much as two off-the-shelf supermarket burgers. Without a doubt, I feel closer to the landscape, the place, and the people that contributed to my sustenance and enjoyment of food. "Sense of community" may be an overused phrase, but when the distance between you as eater and the system of production that feeds you is dramatically shortened, when you feel your own corporal fibers woven into that thread of life, there is a strengthening of the communal bond—a bond that I have now found more joyful and exhilarating than loading my grocery cart from the meat case.

CHAPTER 6
THE FARMER'S COW

Willie Nelson once said, "Dairy farmers are among the hardest workers I know." Having hung around a couple of dozen Connecticut dairy farmers off and on for twenty-five years, I'm inclined to agree. Cows are milked two or three times a day, 365 days a year. It doesn't matter if it's Christmas, your birthday, or ten degrees below zero. Cows don't ever give you a day off.

While hard work might earn dairy farmers a better place in heaven, it hasn't earned them much else these days. According to figures compiled by Robert Wellington, the chief economist for the Northeast region dairy co-op Agri-Mark, Connecticut dairy farmers have made a profit in only nine of seventy-six months ending in February 2009. That's probably why the state has only 157 dairy farms left—down from 663 in 1980—and why the Connecticut legislature passed a short-term dairy bailout bill in its 2009 session.

But sitting in the boardroom of the Farmer's Cow office in Lebanon, Connecticut, one gets a more optimistic impression. Maybe it's the 300 multicolored pushpins stuck in a Connecticut map marking the stores that carry this locally branded milk. Or maybe it's the handmade table fashioned from beautifully finished cedar planks salvaged from a nearby tumbled-down grain silo. Whatever it is, you feel like the Farmer's Cow could be the end of the dairy farmer blues that have been sung in these parts for far too long.

Robin Chesmer is one of six state dairy farmers who make up the

Farmer's Cow, LLC. He's bearded, bespectacled, and stout enough to throw and pin a 1,200-pound heifer in less than thirty seconds. Not that he would, of course. He simply loves his cows too much to ever get rough with them. Chesmer, who with his son Lincoln owns the 700-acre Graywall Farm, explained at some length how attentive they are to the cows' diet, comfort, and happiness. "A cow's stomach is a giant fermentation vat with lots of delicate bacterial flora. You have to give her just the right ratio of grass, protein, and energy." And sounding a bit like an overindulgent parent, Chesmer added, "Cows need nineteen hours a day to just do their own thing. They need to be stress-free." Like all six of his fellow dairypersons, Chesmer told me you will find neither bovine growth hormones (rBGH) nor antibiotics in the Farmer's Cow milk.

But as the Beatles said, "Your lovin' gives me a thrill, but your lovin' don't pay my bills." For all his compassionate husbandry and careful land stewardship, the price Chesmer receives for his milk is determined by the federal milk marketing order, one of the more arcane forms of economic wizardry ever developed by a civilized society. In New England, where the cost of producing milk runs from $18 to $20 per 100 pounds, the farmer is currently receiving only about $13.

"We decided to go ahead with the Farmer's Cow in 2004 because we're in the middle of the one of the largest consumer markets in the world, but we couldn't take advantage of that because we had a faceless product," said Chesmer, referring to the fact that his milk used to be dumped, with nearly every other New England farmer's, into one undifferentiated regional pool. Now, Graywall Farm, along with the other member dairies of the Farmer's Cow—Maple Leaf Farm, Cushman Farm, Fairvue Farm, Hytone Farm, and Fort Hill Farm—collects members' milk into their own pool. Together, they took the courageous step of creating their own brand; they printed their own milk cartons, created some impressive graphics, and even wrote their own song (though it's not destined to be a Grammy winner, you can hear it on their Web site).

Their milk is now available at stores large and small, including some of New England's biggest chain supermarkets.

That a commodity like milk could establish a commercial-scale local identity is just one more symptom of locavore-itis, that near-feverish condition afflicting ever-growing numbers of people who crave a more intimate relationship with their food. And Chesmer and his colleagues share a great deal of culpability for feeding that frenzy. All six farmers and their families have a nonstop schedule of appearances in stores, at farmers' markets, and at festivals around the state to promote their product and educate consumers about cows and farming. "We had a farm tour at Nate Cushman's dairy that drew 600 people," Chesmer told me in disbelief.

While the Farmer's Cow is a dynamic enterprise that gives the consumer a direct connection to Connecticut's farms, it's still not out of the financial woods. The recession has hurt sales because struggling consumers are buying more of the slightly less expensive regional brands. Revenues must be plowed back into the business, postponing any immediate benefit to the farmers. And even though other farmers are clamoring to join the Farmer's Cow, there is still excess capacity among the current six.

THE LAND

Outside of the Farmer's Cow's office window is a landscape to die for—rolling pastures, gently swelling hills, and a barn or two. Losing this beautiful and productive land is ultimately what's at stake. Giving the state's remaining dairy farmers a chance to make a decent living is also on the line. But it all starts with the land.

To extend an old saying: No farmer, no cows; no land, no farmer, no cows; no land, no farmer, no cows, no food, and no humankind—the end. And on it goes in an interconnected web of natural and man-made relationships that have been cultivated in a rough-and-tumble way for thousands of years. Through its ups and downs, in feast and in famine, and in spite of humans' abuses and tendency to career dangerously close to the precipice, the chain has remained unbroken. That is, until the last fifty or so years, when farm- and ranchland came under assault from those with a different set of values.

At some point, growing food and raising animals were no longer considered agricultural land's highest and best use. "It's just a farm," was the dismissive phrase of developers and town officials. "Instead of a bunch of grass with dumb cows on it," these men would say, "I see one thousand new homes, above-ground pools, schools, sewers, soccer fields, and a nearby mall." Such men (I've rarely heard a woman say anything comparable) were considered visionaries in their time. They supposedly saw things that ordinary mortals were blind to. They were lauded for their civic-mindedness, given special seats at Rotary Club luncheons, and recognized with streets named after them in their new subdivisions.

Fortunately, these questionable visionaries and their political sycophants have fallen from favor in many communities. But it has taken a new vision supported by a renewed land ethic to restore agriculture to a standing at least on par with that of developed land. Grass-roots campaigns, sustained public education efforts, and political organizing from the village common to the state legislature have all been necessary to cultivate a land preservation ethic in places where development is a constant challenge to control.

Robin Chesmer wasn't raised on a farm. He came to the United States from England as a boy of seven with little agrarian heritage to draw upon. His interest in farming grew spontaneously from an early and quite natural connection to the soil. Except in Robin's case, the soil was a mere strip of backyard where he nurtured his childhood fantasy of farming with, of all things, Dinky Toys. Across a few square yards of grass and dirt, he assembled miniature farm equipment and plastic livestock. He even "constructed" tiny replicas of New England stone walls from pebbles. "I couldn't wait to get the Sears and Roebuck catalog," he told me, "because they had such a great selection of farm accessories that I imagined one day buying. In my case, I can truly say, my childhood experience had an impact on me today."

A boy's imagination is a powerful thing. I can attest to that. With model replicas of tanks, howitzers, and a couple of hundred plastic soldiers, epic battles raged across the great plains of my sandbox. Fortunately for humanity, I put aside thoughts of global military conquest by the time I was fourteen, but Robin, pursuing a peaceful enterprise with toy plowshares, scaled up to the real thing. By the time he was in his twenties, he had acquired his first thirty-acre farm in Connecticut and a veritable Noah's Ark of real mooing, neighing, and oinking livestock to go with it. His first forays into commercial-scale farming were tentative, supporting himself and his young family with a successful nonfarm retail business. But when a neighboring farmer neared retirement, Robin approached him with an offer to purchase his land. If the farmer had sold the land at its full market price—a number that was getting beyond the reach of area farmers due to encroaching development from Hartford and Norwich—that might have been the end of Robin's dreams. Fortunately for those who favor open, working land over two-acre subdivisions, the retiring farmer was able to sell his "development rights" to the State of Connecticut at the same time he sold his "farming rights" to Robin.

How does that kind of deal work? Say you are the owner of 100 acres of working farmland (actively earning income from an agricultural enterprise): chances are, especially in more developed areas, that the land's market price (or value on the open market for something like housing development) is greater than its value as farmland. The market price minus what area farmers would pay for that land is what's called its development value. When a public agency like the Connecticut Department of Agriculture or a nonprofit land trust buys the development rights, it pays the landowner that value in return for an easement on that land that prevents or severely restricts any development from taking place in perpetuity. The landowner continues to own the land and use it in whatever manner he or she wants—farm it, not farm it, or sell it—but the current and all future owners must abide by the terms of the easement.

Public policy tools like these—formally called a purchase of development rights, or PDR—are what got Robin into dairy farming. A practical vehicle to protect farmland was necessary to marry a wannabe farmer to the land, or to ensure that future farmers would have land available to them to farm. Without that marriage certificate, so to speak, the act of farming could be untenable. And, as in marriage, there is in agriculture what Robin calls "romancing the farm," a love of the land, animals, and the enterprise itself that, when combined with a supportive family and community, can provide someone with the richest and most satisfying life imaginable.

The farmers' passion, rarely expressed in other than a taciturn fashion to the outsider, can be apprehended in the way their eyes assess the landscape, not unlike the way a painter imagines translating that landscape's colors and shapes to a canvas. The farmer will gently manipulate the terrain with tractor and implements, drawing on mental records of other portions of the field, soil types, and drainage. The land and changing light give the farmer his palette. "Doing contours," as Robin called it, "over the fields, alternating hay with corn with fallow earth; finding the right shape and pattern across the slopes is as much an artistic expression as it is a means to control runoff and erosion. There is a blend of art, a desire to be neat and tidy in how you lay down your lines. Watching the cut hay fall behind your tractor is like sitting in the stern of a motorboat watching the wake you're churning up. It's mesmerizing. You immediately notice the change in the color as the drying hay turns from green to yellow. It's as much beauty as business; it's as much art as science." But before he let himself get carried away with the sensuality of farming, Robin emphasized that the reward comes in producing a high-protein feed, and how producing your own feed on the land reduces your imports and makes the farm a self-sufficient operation.

The business note brings us back to the reality of earning a livelihood from the land. It reminds us that no matter how delicious the land looks, you can't eat the scenery. But the interrelationships between the producer and the consumer, the aesthetic and the practical, and the heart and the head are as profoundly important to the farming enterprise as they are to consumer behavior. If a producer operates within the commodity system of food production, processing, and marketing, then there is little need to interact with the consumer because the product is usually sold through a highly structured process that only a few people ever see. However, the farmer, whose profit margin depends on direct marketing—for example, a farmers' market or a local brand identity—must seek the support of the consumer. And capturing that loyalty, especially when the appeal is based on local and sustainable forms of food production, requires something that far exceeds conventional marketing and merchandising practices. It requires that the farmer and those who advocate for a local food system cultivate the sympathies of at least two parts of every person—the part that is a consumer and the part that is a citizen.

The Farmer's Cow did its due marketing diligence. Among other forms of consumer research, the members of the co-operative conducted shopper intercepts in supermarkets to ask consumers questions about their food purchasing choices. They found, for instance, that 84 percent of the respondents would be more likely to purchase dairy products if they knew that would help local dairy farmers. Additionally, respondents indicated they would even pay more to buy local agricultural products. When shown the clever graphics, cute cow pictures, and the "family orientation" photos (generations of overalled, becapped, and smiling farmers) on the carton, consumers also responded favorably. These findings mirror those of similar surveys around the country. When asked if they will buy local farm products when these are identifiable and available, consumer surveys consistently show a 70–90 percent positive rating. But do those consumers follow through when the surveyor is out of sight and the new product is actually on the shelf? Every marketer knows the answer is "no!" There is a huge gap between what people say they will do when asked a series of questions by an enthusiastic, clipboard-toting student earning money for college, and what they actually will do when faced with dozens of choices for a product like milk.

Robin and his colleagues know these things as well, which is why they are relentlessly and creatively promoting the Farmer's Cow in as many intimate, face-to-face venues as they can manage. In one six-month period alone in 2009, they had over twenty major appearances scheduled, each of which drew hundreds and in some cases thousands of people. And that didn't include dozens of smaller events, such as showing up at farmers' markets around the state with a calf or two that "volunteered" to be touched that day by hundreds of eager hands. Granted, some of these promotional activities teeter on the brink of country schmaltz, but there is something going on here that deepens consumer understanding of how farms operate. Without forcing someone to stand knee-deep in a manure pit to develop empathy with the farmer, the exchanges that take place between farmer and nonfarmer have succeeded in partially desanitizing the relationship between us, food, and its source. The Farmer's Cow's commitment to educate the public in a friendly but authentic manner, using a healthy dose of realism, has generated not just a base of loyal shoppers, but also a cadre of well-informed food citizens who then become eager defenders of local farms.

"We're bringing the farm to the public," is the way Robin described it. "They need to meet the farmer and the cow that made the product." These are all things that the growing legions of farmers' market shoppers grasp intuitively, but when it comes to a commodity product like milk, it takes more than a nice shopping experience spent squeezing and sniffing the produce. This is why the Farmer's Cow's six farmers have thrown open their gates to the public. Collectively, they are saying, "We have nothing to hide; you are welcome, and by God, we'll even post directions to our farms on our Web site."

"People have idyllic views about agriculture, but when they come to the farm and see why we do the things we do, they understand," said Robin. While they spare their customers a boot camp experience in farming, the farmers don't water down the realism. The odor of agriculture, the blood-and-guts trauma of birth and death, and the sweat and tears of wresting something profitable from the earth are all honestly revealed. "This is an eye-opening experience for the consumer. They even get excited about how we handle manure."

Consumer education is not limited to on-farm or countryside events; increasingly, the Farmer's Cow is extending into urban areas as well. Robin told me the story of attending a food fundraiser in New Haven. "I found myself talking to a state legislator who told me that she didn't have any dairy farms in her district. The implication was that she didn't have a reason to care about farming. When I told her that the store that sold more of the Farmer's Cow milk than any other store in the state was in her district, her ears perked up. I told her that her constituents really want the Farmer's Cow. Now she's a local agriculture supporter."

The emphasis on expanding the public's understanding of Connecticut agriculture has paid farmers dividends that can be more significant than increased product sales. For many, it has earned them protection of their livelihoods, the retention of their land, and the public's loyalty—loyalty that has been translated into support from policy makers like the one that Robin spoke to. How did this happen? How, in a state that lost a higher percentage of its farmland than any other state in the country in recent years—12 percent from 1997 to 2002 (a pace that if sustained would mean the end of Connecticut's farmland by the year 2040)—did things begin to turn around?

The answers start with the same assumption that the Farmer's Cow has about dairy farming and the consumer: if farmers let consumers see what they are doing, and explain why they are doing it, then people's good sense and reasonableness are likely to inform their choices and actions. If consumers have some personal experience of farming or a particular farmer, they are more likely to choose products made by that farmer or by other local producers. Similarly, we can expect citizens in a democracy to act reasonably, which usually means acting in their self-interest, if they have developed sufficient personal connection to something like farmland and its relation to a necessity like food.

"Save the Land was the start of the movement to save farming in Connecticut," said Robin, referring to a statewide conference held in 1999 at Wesleyan University and sponsored by the Connecticut Food Policy Council. The conference attracted nearly 200 people, who were forced to confront the fact that the state's once-proud agricultural heritage (Connecticut was known as the "provision state" in the Revolutionary War for its role in producing the food that fueled Washington's army) was on a steady course to extinction. After a day of hearing bad news, dire forecasts, and explanations for the current state of affairs, the conference participants agreed to organize around one goal: save Connecticut's farmland.

That was the beginning of what has been a ten-year campaign not only to preserve farmland, but ultimately to enhance the state of agriculture in Connecticut. "At the time of the conference," said Robin, "people had a general appreciation of agriculture, but there has been a very definite shift in attitude since then. People are concerned about what they eat, where their food comes from, and don't want to live in some kind of mass suburbia." If shifts in attitude can be measured by supportive statements from unlikely allies, the words of Bill Purcell, a state Chamber of Commerce leader, are an important bellwether: "[A]cross Connecticut, farmland preservation and open space conservation are essential ingredients in a well-balanced approach to . . . maintaining our quality of life. I urge all of my Chamber of Commerce colleagues to heed the call to keep our farming industry healthy." To have an institution like the Chamber of Commerce, whose main public purpose is just to say no to taxes, endorse farmland preservation is tantamount to the

Republicans issuing a press release extolling the virtues of a Democratic public option health care plan.

This change of heart from business leaders and even home builders was due in part to the most significant organizational outgrowth of the Save the Land conference, namely, the establishment of the Working Lands Alliance (WLA). Within a short period of time WLA would grow to become a coalition of 150 organizations, ranging from the Audubon Society and the Nature Conservancy to the Farm Bureau, Connecticut Department of Agriculture, End Hunger Connecticut, and a host of other farm and environmental organizations. It would soon become the leading voice advocating for the revitalization of the state's previously moribund farmland preservation program. The WLA would largely succeed in accomplishing this task by reminding residents and the state's policy makers that the benefits of farming and farmland extend far beyond their obvious agricultural value. Open space, aesthetics, clean air and water, wildlife habitat, hunting and fishing, historical significance—to say nothing of getting a great local tomato—were all suggested as reasons to preserve farmland and enhance farming. Running up so many pennants on a single flagpole was a powerful way to remind the public of what Europeans like to call the "multifunctionality" of agriculture, by which they mean exactly what the WLA did—that farming and farmland touch nearly every part of the human experience.

This message wasn't lost on the state's policy makers. With slow but steady progress, undergirded by a persistent public education campaign and lobbying effort, WLA gradually wrung concessions out of an at first reluctant state legislature and a hostile governor John Rowland, who saw in farmland only future subdivision sites. Slowly, farmland preservation money reappeared. A farm or two a year would be preserved under the state's PDR program. By the end of the twenty-first century's first decade, well over 50 more farms had been added to the list of 200 preserved before the program stalled in the mid-1990s. Instead of making excuses, Connecticut's political leaders were now confessing that they hadn't done enough. Senator Don Williams, president pro tem of the Connecticut State Senate, said, "Connecticut hasn't invested as much as we need to in farmland preservation. The legislature thinks nothing of putting $100 million into the fuel cell industry; why not agriculture? Why shouldn't the State of Connecticut help agriculture?" By 2005, Williams's pleadings and six years of WLA advocacy were paying off. The Connecticut legislature passed groundbreaking ("ground-saving" might be a better phrase) legislation in the form of the Community Investment Act, which established a $30 real estate transaction fee to be deposited into a fund dedicated to open space, farmland, and historic preservation. The act, which has generated tens of millions of dollars for the fund, also sets aside money for farm viability programs that enable farmers, towns, and nonprofit organizations to expand and develop farm or farm-related businesses. In 2009, the efforts on behalf of Connecticut dairies also paid off. The fee established in the Community Investment Act was raised to $40, a portion of which will be used for at least two years to partially reduce the state's dairy industry's financial loss.

The momentum to save farmland and enhance farming was not limited to the halls of the state capitol building. As a direct outgrowth of the WLA's work, the Connecticut Farmland Trust was formed to fill a niche to protect farms either too small or too specialized to meet the criteria of the state's PDR program. Using private funds and charitable gifts of land, the nonprofit land trust had protected eighteen farms totaling 1,700 acres as of 2009. One of its biggest achievements, however, came in the form of an educational bacchanal called the Celebration of Connecticut Farms and Food that started in 2001. In bringing together the state's best chefs, food, wine, artists, writers, and movie stars under giant tents erected at stunningly beautiful farms, the state's farms and farmland got a boost such as no elected official could ever have conferred. With tickets going for $150 each and corporate sponsorships exceeding $10,000 apiece, the September event has become a "must go" for the state's foodies. And when the likes of Paul Newman, Sam Waterston, and Meryl Streep show up to lend their celebrity status to the cause, well, farming never looked so sexy.

The passion to protect the land has caught fire at the community level as well. The *Hartford Courant* reported: "Of late, residents of many towns have begun to see the value in keeping farms and fields intact rather than turning them into large-lot subdivisions." Citing several towns that combined municipal funds with state and federal money to purchase the development rights to farms within their borders, the *Courant* article went on to say that "it feels like an uptick, especially in farm preservation," attributing the swelling interest in farms to "the amazing growth and popularity of farmers' markets."

Robin Chesmer noted that there are three smaller farms in his community of Lebanon that were negotiating with the Connecticut Farmland Trust (as of 2009) to sell and/or donate easements. In the past, the trust had to scour the landscape far and wide in search of possible deals. Now the deals are beating a path to its door. The Town of Lebanon has hired a full-time planner to focus on farming and farmland issues. And Robin, ever astute to the locus of power and the role of public policy, now serves as a member of the town's planning and zoning commission. The commission's primary goal is to revamp Lebanon's Plan of Development and Conservation to place a heavier emphasis on the role of—guess what?—agriculture.

Is it the dawning of the Age of Aquarius? In Connecticut, anyway (as well as in hundreds of communities across America), there is a growing realization that the community's greatest treasure lies in its topsoil, and that those few inches of fertile matter are all that stand between us and a rather short and brutish life. But that realization hasn't come easily. It was purchased with the loss of hundreds of thousands of acres of prime farmland and the eruption of some of the most hideous developments that anyone has ever seen. With the commitment to public education and advocacy shown by people like Robin Chesmer, Don Williams, the members of the Working Lands Alliance, and thousands of local citizens, the tide has turned.

CHAPTER 7

GOD DIDN'T MAKE NACHOS

The scene inside Primera Iglesia Adventista swung erratically be-tween passive confusion and active chaos. As the crowd of women and children began to swell within the unadorned Austin, Texas, church sanctuary, so did the noise level. Young children, too long held captive by their mothers' firm grips, were temporarily freed to unleash a reign of terror across this little patch of God's kingdom. The soft Spanish chatter of the adults was soon drowned out by the sound of running, screaming children, punctuated by the crash of metal chairs on concrete floors. The pandemonium was brought to a momentary hiatus by a crying child for whom the play had be-come too rough, but after a brief scolding, a dusting off, and a kiss from Mama, the child rejoined the gang of tiny desperadoes. As the roar surpassed its previous decibel levels, the mothers appeared unfazed, and the dime-store portrait of Jesus suspended behind the altar seemed to roll its eyes.

Before the turbulence became unmanageable, Joy Casnovsky, the Austin-based Sustainable Food Center's program director, called out to the day care providers to round up the children and take them to a different room. The food class, known as the Happy Kitchen/la Cocina Alegre™ was about to begin.

Dutifully, the twenty-five or so assembled adult students took their seats. All were Latino, only one was male, and all but three were under forty-five years old. They all came from the lower-income immigrant neighborhood that surrounded the church, an area devoid of decent food stores but rich in junk food outlets. They sat on collapsible metal chairs that only those doing penance for multiple sins should have to endure. The rows formed a series of shallow arcs around a ten-foot-wide cutout in the wall that separated the sanctuary from the church's kitchen. Three instructors and a couple of their older daughters stood in the kitchen looking through the opening at the audience, who in turn stared back at them as if watching a wide-screen TV.

Maria Tinoco, the lead facilitator and a former student in the class, held up a bowl of sugar and a teaspoon. She began to spoon the sugar into a clear glass container, and as if on cue all twenty-five students began to count along: "Uno, dos, tres . . . nueve, diez, once." "Once!" shouted Maria, telling everyone that a twelve-ounce can of cola contains eleven teaspoons, or forty-four grams, of pure sugar. Several participants squinched up their noses in disgust. I could feel my own lips purse as my tongue reflexively scrubbed the imagined gunk from the roof of my mouth. While the audience members were generally slimmer than most people I would encounter during my four days in Austin, the fear of diabetes hung like a black shroud over the room. Sugar was public enemy number one.

Paula, a notably svelte woman, told me, "My father has diabetes and most of my family has high cholesterol. Though they are all fat, they don't want to change. I don't want to be like that." The poor dietary role models offered by her family motivated Paula to attend the six Happy Kitchen classes, each of which gave her the knowledge to avoid the slippery slope to diabetes and the degraded health conditions prevalent in her family. "I don't drink sodas and my children don't either. But my sister drinks four sodas a day! I only cook fish and chicken, no red meat, and only brown rice, no white rice. And I carefully read food labels."

After scaring the audience with her graphic demonstration of the evils of soft drinks, Maria offered aqua fresca as a healthy alternative. Using club soda and 100 percent fruit juice or fresh fruit such as strawberries, then locally in season, she concocted a drink that had the refreshing effervescence of soda but only the natural sweetness of fruit. The audience loved it.

A tripod stand was placed stage right supporting a "Mi Pirámide" USDA food pyramid poster in Spanish. Jovita, another instructor, picked up where Maria had left off by pointing at the chart and underlining what you shouldn't and should eat. She reinforced the lesson by passing around some food packages, soda cans, and bottles with their nutrition labels intact. Reading and understanding these labels is a critical emphasis of the Happy Kitchen. As one participant would later tell me, "Knowledge is power," and when armed with a better understanding of these labels, the participants expressed a greater confidence in their ability to make healthy food choices.

I realized how deficient my own knowledge was when I started perusing the nutrition label on the empty soda can. I had, of course, assumed that my graduate degree was more than sufficient to enable me to decipher something as simple as a nutrition label. But until Maria's vivid teaspoon demonstration, I hadn't been able to visualize grams of sugar. Now that I could, it became clear how little of it I should be consuming. Based on surveys that the Happy Kitchen conducts for every session, almost 60 percent of the participants have only a high school diploma or less. I concealed my chagrin when I realized that most of the participants at this point probably knew as much as, or perhaps more than, I did about healthy eating.

I find that nearly every time I give a presentation about food, I'll get a mix of questions and comments like the following: "Why don't people know how to eat right?" "What we need is more food education in our schools." "Why not bring back home economics?" "Why do we need nutrition education? Eating is as normal as breathing, walking, and drinking water. We don't offer education for them."

Others, including me, will say, "Society and the food industry are the problem." "Fast food and bad food are cheap and prevalent, especially in lower-income and underserved communities (food deserts)." And conversely, "Healthy food is more expensive and not prevalent in many communities." "We have become a go-go, nonstop nation of soccer moms and football dads; convenience is all that matters and no one eats together anymore."

From advocates for locally and organically produced food I often hear: "People just need to 'get in touch' with their food and where it comes from." "People need to garden. Everyone who gets their hands in the dirt develops a better appreciation for food." "People have choices. They can either spend their money buying two pairs of Nikes and cable television, or they can buy organic [expensive] food."

There's some truth to all of these comments. The industrial food system and our market economy have done an admirable job of disengaging us from our sustenance and, in the process, separating food and agriculture from human and environmental health. They have been supported by a media and advertising apparatus that have succeeded in persuading us to do things to our health that sometimes appear masochistic, like making us believe that we can derive eating pleasure only from a 1,500-calorie triple-decker burger laced with cheese and bacon. Our public schools have done little to counter the messages of the food industry. Effective food education is still a rarity, and even when their impossibly tight funding allows some room for new initiatives, public school programs are no match for the budgets and wizardry of America's marketing moguls.

As enlightened as many of us have become about the public health menace of obesity, why do so many of us choose to eat the wrong things when we have the means and access, at least in most cases, to eat the right things? When over 60 percent of Americans are overweight or obese, can we truly lay all the blame at the feet of the food system and not hold the individual accountable?

My travels take me through far too many airports where the large number of overweight and obese families waddling down the concourses makes me cry out in frustration. There are moments, I confess, when I feel a visceral revulsion at this parade of undulating flesh. The parents are barely able to conceal their rolls of fat beneath baggy and flagrantly branded windbreakers and oversize sweatpants. They are leading tragically obese children who are sipping Coke from their quart-size McDonald's cups. Such families, of course, use the moving walkway, spurning the few minutes of exercise they might get if they chose to walk the 300 feet between gates. Likewise, portly businessmen, their amply tailored Brooks Brothers suit jackets failing to adequately cover their distended bellies, pace back and forth in a state of hyperagitation. Their red faces are etched with stress as they speak into the airy nothing, or maybe it's the Bluetooth surgically attached to their ears. In one hand they clutch their iPod, in the other a double-bacon cheeseburger.

America on the move in public places, especially at the agonizingly slow pace of the painfully heavy, depresses me. My posture crumbles as I slump into my chair and exhale an insuppressible sigh of grief. Surrounded by Cinnabons and Taco Bells, I can't muster an appetite for anything more than cottage cheese. In this fevered state, I begin to imagine that day in an airport when a true emergency occurs, when a band of terrorists has broken through TSA's otherwise indomitable line of defense and threatens to exterminate the terminal's inhabitants. I can visualize how the chaotic scene will unfold. The announcement comes over the public address system that the airport is in a state of red alert. Everybody should proceed as fast as possible to the nearest exit. Families are desperately clinging to one another as they struggle to reach any open doorway. But the huffing and puffing gets the better of the panicked fathers, who collapse with chest pains to the ground. The few agile and slim members of the crowd are able to slip away, sprinting to freedom across the vast expanse of tarmac. But the others, the overwhelming majority, those whom the Centers for Disease Control have deemed at risk, are left gasping, drenched in sweat, piled against one another like a massive car accident on the New Jersey Turnpike. Unable to fight or flee, Americans are undone from within, making themselves easy targets for those who hate us.

Besides staying out of airports, is there another way for me to resolve my nightmare? Yes, the private marketplace, which has little regard for the public interest, must change itself, and must be changed by others—government, writers, activists—so that the populace has the opportunity to make better dietary choices. But how will individuals find the strength and the will to change their own behavior? After all, the decision to eat healthily or not ultimately rests in no one's hands but our own.

Listening to dozens of women from the Happy Kitchen tell their stories gave me a clear idea of how and why people make changes that can literally save their lives. For Sharon Ellerby, a middle-aged African American woman living in Austin, the path to a healthy lifestyle was revealed in her teens. Like many people I spoke with, her decision to change her diet initially sprang from ill health. In her case it was childhood asthma; and in the case of her grandmother, who raised Sharon, it was a stroke that felled the sixty-seven-year-old woman, who was overweight but otherwise solid as a rock. Grandma recovered and lived to the towering age of eighty-nine, but only with Sharon's assistance as a devoted and live-in caregiver.

"Now I'm in control!" Sharon told me over coffee at the Blue Dahlia café in east Austin. Her distinct note of triumph was one I would hear time and again, stated both explicitly and implicitly by the Happy Kitchen participants. In Sharon's case, control meant that she would play a primary role in nursing her grandmother back to health, which she did by taking charge of her diet. But control also meant that in the process of helping others, Sharon and her peers were also taking control of their own lives.

"My grandmother was a great cook. She was always frying up chicken and selling it right out of her house. And if people were hungry and needed to eat, they knew that Grandma's house was the place to go [for a free meal]." This kind of generosity and compassion rubbed off on Sharon. Her care for her incapacitated grandmother would translate later into social service jobs with HIV/AIDs programs, the Austin Housing Authority, and eventually as a facilitator/instructor with the Happy Kitchen.

But during the time she cared for her grandmother, Sharon was unable to work. Without insurance, she suddenly realized that her health, as well as her grandmother's, was now in her own hands. She turned to a changed diet to prevent illness, and to "natural healing" to cure herself when illness couldn't be prevented. For her, "natural" meant those things that come from the earth, made by God, and untainted by man-made chemicals. Though religious, Sharon does not invoke faith, scripture, or dogma in telling her story. She's grounded in a low-key but deeply spiritual reserve born of experience and caring for others.

Though her grandmother was a positive role model, in that she taught Sharon compassion and a love of food, especially in a cultural and community context, her grandmother was also a negative role model, in that her sudden decline in health was caused in large part by unhealthy food preparation methods. At the very least, Sharon did not want to end up like her grandmother. "Fear is a motivator," she acknowledged, and after she became a Happy Kitchen facilitator she discovered she shared that motivating force with others. Speaking of the participants in her classes, she said, "I could see the fear in their eyes. They didn't want to end up in a wheelchair." (Fear of succumbing to chronic illness and becoming dependent on others were major factors in almost everyone's food stories).

While it might have been fear that initially drove Sharon to act, it was innate curiosity combined with a belief in her own potential that sent her on a voyage of self-education. Through reading books, searching the Internet, and talking to others, she became more confident in her own abilities to manage her diet, her health, and herself. And when she came to the Happy Kitchen for the first time as a participant in 2004, she was eager for even more knowledge. Her eagerness paid off, she told me, with a major weight loss. "Before the class I wore a size 16. A few weeks after completing the six-week session, I was wearing a size 10."

Whether in sickness or in health, the nurturing instinct is alive and kicking. Of course, one can say that this is a traditional female role that is as old as Eve—the dedicated spouse, the nursing mother, the dutiful daughter/granddaughter/sister. But somehow the revelations about diet and health, especially over the course of the twenty-first century—the soaring rates of juvenile and adult onset diabetes, increasing food allergies, food safety scares, and a host of environmental threats—have given a new urgency and perhaps a new meaning to the role of nurturing, a role that men, of course, think they share equally, but in fact still leave largely to women.

Susana Trujeque-Cooper came to Texas from Mexico, where her mother cooked traditional foods such as enchiladas, beans, and rice. "I learned to cook from my mama, who taught me to cook with love." When I asked her to tell me what she meant by cooking with love, Susana explained that her mother didn't rush around the kitchen trying to slap a meal together in haste in order to meet the family's scheduling demands. Her mother saw meal preparation as way to spend what we might call quality time with both her food and her family. She moved deliberately around the kitchen, handled the tortillas with care, seasoned the dishes with attention to her own nuance and style. "This was her way of showing love for her family," said Susana. Without knowing it, Susana's mother shared her approach to cooking with the Slow Food movement, which practices its relationship to food to the beat of a rhythm that fits the strides of season and the exigencies of place—a pacing that is suited to the natural tempo of the human body and the natural pulse of the senses.

But there was something missing from her mother's cooking. No matter how much love she brought to each day's meal preparation, Susana's mother lacked knowledge of the connections between each dish's ingredients, overall diet, and health. "I used to think that all breads, oils, and juice were the same until I took my first Happy Kitchen class five years ago," said Susana. The classes would plant seed after seed in her fertile mind, and they have never stopped bearing fruit. "I use whole wheat pasta now and only canola or olive oil to cook with. I'm serving more variety of foods but smaller serving sizes." And, with her dark eyes widening to the size of cucumber slices, she told me in a state of near rapture how to make her favorite drink, orange juice combined with pineapple juice and fresh spinach leaves. "Spinach?" I asked, taken aback. "Yes, it comes out green, but it's delicious!"

Within her own household she has had ample opportunity to test her recipes for love and knowledge. "My husband is an American person [in this case, African American] and loves his meat but not vegetables." Lowering her voice to almost a whisper, she confessed to me that she sometimes mixes tofu in with his meat, which he has so far failed to detect. But her bigger challenge is with her two daughters, nine and twelve, not because they don't like healthy food, but because their father, Susana's ex-husband, shares custody. "My daughters eat very healthy with me, but not when they are with their father. He takes them out to fast food places a lot." This clearly frustrates Susana, who feels that her daughters are getting mixed messages, but even worse, her diligent efforts to feed and teach her daughters well are being undermined. Nevertheless, she believes her daughters know what is right and have developed a taste for a wide variety of foods, including fresh fruits and vegetables. She added with pride that on Sunday, the day that her daughters go to their father, "they often ask me to make a healthy lunch for them to take to school on Monday because they don't like school lunch."

Susana's challenges brought back some unpleasant memories of my own. As the newly divorced father of a five- and a twelve-year-old, I suddenly realized I was now responsible for preparing meals for my children and myself at least three days per week. For reasons that I could not explain as well then as Susana can now, I categorically refused to take my children to McDonald's, et al., a practice that my "ex" was not willing to give up. While my food knowledge at that time was meager and my kitchen skills pitiful, I at least had a general idea of what was healthy. My theory was more or less sound, but my practice was appalling. Since I was a good gardener, our dinners were often built around a recent harvest, which was great, but when my collard greens came out looking like slurry of decomposed grass clippings, and my ex was serving up meatloaf and mashed potatoes smothered in gravy, followed by apple pie à la mode, it was not surprising that my children would often say of my meals, "Mom doesn't make us eat this stuff!"

Though my children didn't recognize it at the time, I was trying to demonstrate what Susana calls love. And, just as she noted, love without knowledge can have unfortunate consequences. But how, where, and from whom does one gain this knowledge? If our parents don't have it perfectly right or there isn't another adult figure available to teach us, where do we turn? During my middle school days in the mid-1960s, all the boys took wood shop and all the girls took home economics. By the time my younger sisters reached middle school, the dark curtain of sexism was partially lifted and wood shop and home economics were co-ed. Not that either course was worth much, especially by today's standards (my pump lamp soon found its way to the kindling box and my sisters' brownies were suitable only as hockey pucks), but at least the public school system subscribed to the belief that it had some responsibility to prepare young people with practical life skills. As schools slipped ever deeper into financial holes as a result of local taxpayers who only believed (and only barely) in the "three R's," they would start to eliminate "nonessential" programs like music, art, drivers' education, and, of course, wood shop and home economics. As a result, today's young people graduate from public schools not knowing how to use a hammer or a whisk.

"If we don't know how to do something," Susana told me, "we

must learn; if we already know how, we must share." When I asked her how such solid wisdom might be put into practice, she pointed out that "we eat American food because that is our culture, and we don't have a lot of knowledge about the consequences of eating that food. We only think about taste, not about saturated fats; or we only think about calories, not nutrient content, which is why we think we're doing fine when we drink lots of diet sodas. We're also rushing everywhere, and we don't take time to prepare food and eat meals together."

No doubt these are sentiments that everyone, from Slow Food's founder, Carlo Petrini, to Chez Panisse's Alice Waters, would share (Susana was not familiar with either name). But few food leaders like Susana would have emerged from their state of powerlessness and ignorance without assistance. The power to choose may be something we're born with, but power unaided by knowledge is a weak muscle indeed.

"I have the power to make the right choice," said Susana, "because of the knowledge I gained from the Happy Kitchen. I know others don't yet have that knowledge which is why I try to share it." I reminded her that she had told me that her children didn't like the food they received at school, and wondered if she had ever tried to do something about that. "Yes, I have gone to school meetings and told the officials how poor the quality of the food is." Then her eyes went into cucumber slice mode again: "I wouldn't have spoken up at school if wasn't for the Happy Kitchen." Susana's story illustrates how education can empower people to make changes not only in their own lives, but in the wider community as well.

Joy Casnovsky and Valeria Morrow (Val is the Happy Kitchen's program coordinator) have just come off a twelve-hour day. It's 9:00 p.m. and they are chilling out over cold beers and a shared plate of quesadillas. But one beer each is all they allow themselves since they start all over again promptly at 8:15 the following morning. As the program's only two staff members, they spend their long days planning fourteen six-week classes every year, coordinating forty facilitators (though paid only a stipend for their work, the facilitators are the Happy Kitchen's secret weapon), and driving around Austin's crowded roadways in ninety-three-degree heat to procure all the paper, pencils, and tofu each class will need.

Both women are modest and thoughtful, deflecting my offered credit and not wanting to overstate their program's achievements. "Unfortunately," reflected Joy, "too many folks want a quick fix. Changing dietary habits is not quick by any means. Yes, people start to make remarkable changes while enrolled in our program. However, the sessions are not a pill to be taken, and *poof*—you are healthy."

Measuring the success of such programs is a tricky business. The Sustainable Food Center (the Happy Kitchen's parent organization) is participating in a University of Texas study designed to assess the longer-term impact of the Happy Kitchen course on its participants. Joy and Val carefully survey all their students to determine if the community's lower-income population—the program's primary target—is being served, and also to identify the program's short-term impacts.

For the most recent set of eight sessions, over 60 percent of the 114 participants who completed the survey (225 participated in at least one class) identified themselves as from a low- to lower-middle-income household, with 32 percent of the total coming from households with less than $15,000 in annual income. Overall, 15 percent are African American, 73 percent are Hispanic, and, as expected, 95 percent are women.

Perhaps most interesting from a numbers point of view is the percentage of participants who attribute significant changes in their food selection and eating behavior to the Happy Kitchen. Anywhere from 80 to 97 percent of the respondents said, among other things, that they now use nutrition labels to make healthier food choices, eat more fresh fruits and vegetables, and buy lower-fat dairy products and leaner sources of protein. More specifically, participants commented that they are now "buying 1% milk" and "choosing fresh veggies over canned or frozen." One respondent wrote that she "got rid of the unhealthy food and actually lost 10 pounds!" and another, "I learned how to take care of the health of my family."

With results like these, you'd think Joy and Val would be strutting about the café like a couple of peacocks in full feather. As a male of the species, that's exactly what I'd be doing. But as Jim Hightower said in one of his more appropriate barnyard metaphors, "It may be the rooster that crows, but it's the hen that delivers the goods." Joy and Val do the work, quietly report the results, and then set about the task of making things work even better.

Joy is professional and cautious to a fault, her acknowledgements of success also containing their own critique. "I believe that part of what the Happy Kitchen does is makes eating healthy more fun and achievable. Most people are not enthusiastic about eating healthy and losing weight because the connotation around healthy food is that it's going to be a bunch of rabbit food, or it won't taste good, or their children or husband won't touch it." To keep their participation levels up, she and Val confess, they occasionally resort to "bribery." Of the 225 participants noted above, only 125 attended at least four classes, the minimum required to receive the Happy Kitchen's graduation certificate. "We recently started giving the graduates a copy of our 252-page recipe book, where before we would charge $10 for it," remarked Val. They also give away a bag of food to each participant at the end of the class that contains most of the ingredients from that class's instructional meal. At another class I attended, the instructor had asked how many people had tried the dish they had learned about the week before. Almost 90 percent raised their hands. "The book and food definitely give people an incentive to keep coming back, but also serve to reinforce the lessons," said Val.

In spite of ample evidence that the Happy Kitchen is doing more things correctly and effectively to rein in America's collective eating disorder than just about anyone else, their apparent success begs the question of why the program isn't much bigger, or why there aren't more of them. Some of the answers came from the Sustainable Food Center's executive director for four years, Ronda Rutledge. Poised, friendly, and a consummate fund-raiser, Ronda heads a nonprofit organization that has developed a highly integrated and respected model of regional food system action. An organization involved in many activities, from empowering children and adults to grow their own food to supporting farmers' markets to influencing local food policy, the Sustainable Food Center stands out as one of those rare agencies that understands that there are many dots that need to be connected in order to secure a just and sustainable supply of food for all. And it connects those dots very well.

When we spoke, Ronda had just secured a four-acre donation of land in the heart of Austin where the Sustainable Food Center planned to construct its own facility (at the time it had twelve staff people crammed into a leased, bulging-at-the-seams office building) complete with offices, classrooms, a large teaching kitchen, and outdoor gardens. All of this would come to fruition only if Ronda and her colleagues completed a $2.5-million capital campaign. "Our programs are always struggling for funding," said Ronda, "and now we have the opportunity for this new facility that we simply can't pass up. There's a lot of pressure all around."

The size and diversity of Ronda's workload and the many fund-raising demands placed on the center are not meant to imply that the center lacks interest in any one of its hungry programs that must be fed, including the Happy Kitchen. They are simply an acknowledgement of the enormous burdens that change-oriented organizations like the center face, and even more importantly, recognition of the need to sustain a balanced portfolio of programs. But still, with the gravity of the obesity epidemic threatening to undo the nation's health, shouldn't programs like the Happy Kitchen become as prevalent as bluebonnets in a Texas meadow?

Joy and Val provided part of the answer. Since 2006 the Happy

Kitchen has worked closely with Community Food Alliance in Palm Beach County, Florida, providing start-up training and technical assistance and ongoing consultation. While not an official franchise, the Florida program has used most of the Happy Kitchen's methods and materials, paying, by agreement, for these services. A similar group based in Pinehurst, North Carolina, recently contracted for program development services as well. Though this group already had a nutrition education program, it felt it was too "bookish" and wanted something more hands-on like the Happy Kitchen.

Joy, Val, and Ronda all sense there is a potentially big market for their program across the country, but how to package it as a product that can be purchased by other small and underfunded nonprofit organizations is a bit daunting. Selling yourself on a scale that's large enough to replicate the program professionally and effectively while earning sufficient revenue constitutes new but necessary territory for many nonprofits. Nevertheless, the Happy Kitchen is putting together a business plan to do just that.

Obviously, a couple of additional staff people would enable the Happy Kitchen to explore more of these options, continue to refine the quality of its program, and modestly expand its efforts in the Austin area. But Joy posited that a bigger impact could be had in less time if the Austin Independent School District adopted the program as a core component of its overall curriculum. If every high school student went through the Happy Kitchen curriculum for one six-week segment, one could reasonably project a sea change in a generation's dietary health accompanied by a concomitant drop in the nation's collective body mass index. "But with school districts cutting physical education, foreign languages, and the arts," Joy pessimistically asserted, "I don't think they are likely to adopt a system-wide food curriculum anytime soon."

Though the times may not augur well for deep, system-wide change of a broad institutional nature, the Happy Kitchen keeps humming along, pollinating one flower at a time. Gloria Lopez told me how the program has allowed her to get her diabetes under control by teaching her to modify her diet. She's also the caregiver for her husband and a twelve-year-old granddaughter, who often attends the classes with Gloria. Among other ways, they apply their new food knowledge to their nightly television viewing by dissecting and sometimes ridiculing junk food commercials, especially those for fast food restaurants.

When Maria Tinoco moved to Texas from Mexico, she went from 130 pounds to 168 pounds in three months. "It was American food, especially fast food, that did it," she told me. With her own force of will and the knowledge gained in the Happy Kitchen, Maria returned to her "Mexican weight" and is now helping her peers navigate a similar course to a healthy lifestyle.

Pat Zimmerman, seventy-eight, who by her own admission may have been the oldest participant in the Happy Kitchen, is determined to beat the odds that a bad set of cholesterol genes bestowed on her. She told me she's eating better as "an act of rebellion against the threat of a debilitating illness simply because I want to see my grandchildren grow up." So far, the recipes and techniques she has learned from the two sets of classes she's completed—including fish and vegetarian dishes, as well as the use of herbs and spices for flavor—are allowing her hope to come true. (She's also contemplating taking the facilitator's training.)

Belle Smith, forty-three, doesn't see the Happy Kitchen merely as a pathway to healthier eating: for her it's been gateway to a whole new lifestyle. The wake-up call came three years ago when she was diagnosed as pre-diabetic. "I never really cooked before the Happy Kitchen. I ate out at fast food restaurants all the time." She holds a bachelor's degree and an important administrative position in the Austin Community College system, but Belle readily admits that until her "medical awakening," her career came first. She often found herself working fifteen-hour days, sometimes until midnight, and letting everything else in her life, particularly her health, slide. "It's not the level of [a person's] education that matters [when it comes to diet and health], it's your priorities. Because of the encouragement and knowledge I got from the Happy Kitchen I made choices that allowed me to lose weight, start exercising, work less, do community volunteer work, and even get a social life." She added with a chuckle, "I can't tell you how good I felt when my eight-year-old niece asked me, 'Auntie, did you lose weight?'" There are other ripple effects from Belle's changed lifestyle. On the day we had our conversation, she had an appointment to meet with the college's food vending service to discuss the introduction of more healthy options in the cafeteria.

And then there is Dorothy Morrison, who somehow embodied all the hopes and challenges of the women I met. On the one hand, she fit every negative stereotype that our snarly society has dreamed up—a thirty-seven-year-old black woman who was overweight, a single mother of five children ages four to eighteen, and living in public housing. On the other hand, she was a woman who was searching daily for every resource she could find to make as much success as possible from the cards that were dealt her as well as the ones she had dealt to herself.

Her early years consisted of moving around a lot, living with friends and relatives, and often being hungry. As a guest in households that already had too many mouths to feed, "you got what's left over if you got anything at all." She eventually landed in Oakland, California, where she lived with and learned how to cook from her blind grandfather, who had lost his eyesight in a defense industry accident. "My grandfather needed help, and I was naturally curious, so he would teach me everything I asked him, including how to cook."

She admits her first encounter with cuisine was a disaster. "My sister and I put a whole chicken in a boiling pot of water for a couple of hours. It was a mess." But Dorothy's love of cooking and her grandfather's lessons gave her some basic competency in the kitchen. Like that of so many others, however, the daily menu was heavy on fried chicken and other fatty foods, and light on fresh produce. And when she became a mother, she confessed, preparing healthy meals became a strain. "When you're stuck in an unhealthy eating habit for your whole life, it's hard to make a permanent change. It takes a lot of commitment. And when you have five kids, all with different appetites, and I'm tired and stressed out at the end of day, well, they tend to get what they want. That's when it becomes all about convenience." She says one of her sons is obese, and it was partly out of concern for him that she decided to enroll in the Happy Kitchen program.

"They taught me how to make broccoli taste good—without smothering it in cheese," Dorothy told me with a laugh. "I smelled rosemary for the first time and learned to love cilantro. I discovered that I could bake chicken with herbs, and it would have plenty of flavor." She was given simple ideas like the use of colors—the more variety of color on the plate, the more likely you have a balanced and healthy meal. She was introduced to new and healthier twists on old foods, like fresh tomatoes rather than canned. She learned how to read nutrition labels, a skill that she now practices with her children when they go grocery shopping together. "I make them read the labels on cereal boxes so that we buy the ones with the lowest sugar content."

Dorothy made progress, the family was having healthy dinners together, and she lost weight. But with the gains came setbacks. Though she does less frying now, she can't give up immersing those chickens in fatty oils. Nacho chips covered in cheese is still her favorite dish. And she gained back the weight that she had lost while taking the Happy Kitchen classes. Dorothy is a woman with a sweet and gentle nature, a deep abiding faith in God, and an active commitment to the housing project's Christian Women's Job Corps. She works part-time for the Housing Authority of the City of Austin trying to keep young kids out of gangs. Yet her battle to feed herself and others well is continually undermined by a mass food culture that is telling her to do otherwise. She fully acknowledges that what she knows is right is always under assault by the demands of her children and a life on the brink of poverty. Dorothy also knows that losing the battle involves much more than just succumbing to the occasional bucket of KFC. She knows that it's her health and that of her children that are at stake.

"The Happy Kitchen gave me confidence that made me feel more positive as a mom," said Dorothy. "It empowered me to be able to make healthy dinners for my children, and seeing them start to like vegetables gave me more confidence." But she gives her spiritual partner just as much credit. "I always count on the Lord to help me think clearly. Eating healthy has a lot to do with knowing God. Our body is a temple, as the saying goes. After all, God didn't make nachos. He created fruits that grow from the trees and vegetables that grow from the ground. He created cows and chickens, but not the lard to fry them in." There was a long, almost prayerful pause and a searching glance upward. "I seek the willpower to use the knowledge, and I ask for the strength and willpower to make other changes in my life."

CHAPTER 8
HEALTHY SCHOOLS
GROW HEALTHY KIDS

"There needs to be one place in society where children feel that their needs come first. . . . In American society today, schools are the only option. That's why every aspect of school food matters so much," according to Marion Nestle, Paulette Goddard Professor in the Department of Nutrition, Food Studies, and Public Health at New York University. The lessons of Austin's the Happy Kitchen strongly support the notion that it's never too late to learn new ways of eating and cooking. Adults will, of course, be motivated to learn by an entirely different set of reference points than children. Whether they are moving into the position of parent or primary caregiver for the first time, faced with a sudden medical threat, or have finally absorbed the nearly omnipresent messages of healthy eating, grown-ups can and do change for the better. But like many things in life—learning a new language comes to mind—there are some mountains that are best climbed when you're young. As I can personally attest, learning to develop a taste for broccoli would have been far easier as a child than going through the process of radically altering my taste buds at the age of forty.

And then there is the issue of efficiency. As the Happy Kitchen amply illustrates, it takes a lot of work to reach a few hundred adults every year compared to the relative ease with which the program might be taught to every school-age child in Austin. But we Americans favor the short-term approach over the long-term, and let the devil take tomorrow. In Santa Fe, New Mexico, the public school system is attempting to take the devil by the horns with several approaches, including a program known as Cooking with Kids. The point the program's administrators wish to prove is that learning to eat healthy food is something we should all begin to do in our early years. If we can educate the palate and the mind at, say, the age of ten, we will be far better equipped to avoid the scourge of diet-related illnesses at the age of fifty.

"Would you like some salad, my sweetie?" was how Margo Jimenez, a nine-year school food service veteran, affectionately greeted the first wave of third graders coming through the cafeteria line at Alvord Elementary School in Santa Fe, New Mexico. A native of Puerto Rico, Ms. Jimenez is one of 110 Santa Fe school food service employees who prepare and serve lunch to almost 13,000 students every school day in the district's twenty-seven schools. While the job of food service worker requires skills such as meal assembly, food safety and sanitation, and administration, the most important skill just may be that of promoting healthy food. On this particular day the Alvord cafeteria salad bar contained a mix of greens, carrots, cucumbers, and broccoli. Children could choose also from grapes and orange slices and, of course, the all-time local favorite, Frito pie (baked red chile, beans, ground beef, and Fritos). The fruit and salad are not always the children's first choice, but Ms. Jimenez's gentle coaxing usually means that most children end up with one serving each of fruit and vegetables on their plate.

If obesity is one of the most serious health problems facing today's children, then Ms. Jimenez's job may be one of the most important in America. As any parent knows, preparing children to avoid the temptations of foods high in sugar, salt, and fat—and encouraging them to eat their vegetables—can be tough work. Alvord's principal, Betsy Ellvinger, an educator for fifteen years, says, "I see more obesity now than I used to." She knows how important nutrition and health are to parents, noting that she sometimes receives five calls per day from parents about the school's food.

Recently she had to allay the fears of one parent who was very upset when she heard the false rumor that Alvord was going to suspend the operation of its salad bar.

Judy Jacquez is the director of Santa Fe's School Food Service Department, which means that she oversees a large and complex operation whose mission is bigger than its budget. "Just by having healthy food [such as fruits, salad bars, low-fat milk] available, kids will select it, but we need to expand its availability to all our schools," she said, referring to programs such as the introduction of the salad bar at Alvord. But the more fundamental task for Jacquez is putting good food on the plates of Santa Fe students without overspending her budget. Among these students, 7,100 qualify for the federal Child Nutrition Program's free or reduced-price lunch. These lunches, along with breakfasts for 2,500 students every day, are meals that lower-income children and their families depend on: without them, many children would go hungry. And as every teacher knows, children who are distracted by hunger pangs cannot learn.

Since the health and well-being of children are so important, in Santa Fe parent volunteers, private nonprofit organizations, and government agencies have stepped forward with an array of innovative services to augment existing school nutrition efforts. These include assistance from other parts of the Santa Fe school system, such as the Office of Student Wellness, directed by Tita Gervers. Under her direction, Santa Fe is addressing childhood obesity by supporting a healthy school food service program, ensuring that school vending machines contain only healthy food options, including water, 100 percent fruit juice, and trail mix, and enlisting the participation of school nurses, who play a vital role in nutrition education.

Outside of the school system, Craig Mapel of the New Mexico Department of Agriculture is brokering deals between New Mexico farmers and schools in a program called Farm to School. In Santa Fe he works with Betsy Torres of the Santa Fe Public Schools to put locally produced apples, peaches, apricots, lettuce, and watermelons on the cafeteria trays. Today, thirteen of New Mexico's school districts, which collectively serve over 200,000 students—two-thirds of the state's public school students—are participating in Farm to School.

Improving the quality of school food is one critical step down the road to healthier eating, but most food education experts agree that serving good food in the cafeteria must be supported by learning in the classroom. Because sitting children down in front of nutrition textbooks or computer screens to learn how to eat healthily is far less effective than hands-on cooking experience, Santa Fe has adopted a national food education model called Cooking with Kids (CWK). Developed by former Santa Fe chefs Lynn Walters and Jane Stacey, CWK brings food and its history, culture, and preparation directly to the students. On any given day, a CWK food educator will wheel a cart, complete with a two-burner hot plate, griddle, plates, cooking utensils, and food, into a Santa Fe classroom. Since the food represents a particular place or season, students will read about its history, learn how and where it's grown, and also gain important information about its nutritional value. The children then wash their hands carefully, put on aprons, and prepare a meal.

A salad-tasting exercise for second and third graders is one example of how young children can cultivate their senses at the same time they cultivate a taste for vegetables. Curious but quiet, the students are divided into four groups (they are still relatively obedient at this age) and given several kinds of lettuce and red cabbage from a local farm, and sprouts that were grown in the classroom. They are encouraged to taste each ingredient separately and to discuss how each one compares to the other. They are taught to let their thoughts and words reveal the experience of their senses—sight, taste, smell, and touch. While there is some discussion of health and nutrients, one will not hear the dreaded phrase "It's good for you" spoken in a CWK classroom, nor will one witness the infantilization of food ("One day Mr. Cabbage and Miss Lettuce were picked from their garden and became good friends in Mrs.

McGillicuty's salad bowl"). The source of the food is discussed, which in this case is a nearby organic farm. A letter from the farmer is read to the students that describes the farm while sharing some of the history of the family that runs it (on other occasions students may take a field trip to the Santa Fe Farmers' Market or even have a farmer visit them in the classroom). Once their impressions are recorded, the volunteers help them to combine the ingredients in a bowl and drizzle the contents with salad dressing. And with a decorum rarely seen among children of this age by this writer, they sit down politely to enjoy the salad together.

According to Walters, "When people participate in food preparation they are naturally more interested in it." This is clearly borne out by the enthusiastic responses of children, who have said such things as: "I like Cooking with Kids because we make good food," "I liked that the pizza had different kinds of vegetables," "I love to cook. I make tamales at home with my mom," "I liked chopping the garlic best," "I love it. Can we have the recipe?" and "The chile rocks!" What's happening with CWK is that children are developing a love of cooking and a taste for quality ingredients as well as varied cuisines, all of which may lead to long-term positive health outcomes.

By the numbers, CWK annually serves about 4,500 Santa Fe elementary school students, each of whom participates in eleven food classes over the course of the full school year. While the program doesn't reach all of the city's schools and students, almost every elementary school student will receive at least one round of CWK classes somewhere between the second and sixth grade. The total cost for one student to go through the full-year program is $90. Is it worth it? According to figures from the Center for Disease Control and Prevention, New Mexico spends at least $325 million a year on health care costs to treat obesity-related illnesses. If every fourth grader in New Mexico participated in CWK, that would cost all the state's school districts about $3 million per year, or 1 percent of the annual obesity cost.

While it's reasonable to expect that such an investment would yield at least a tenfold return through a reduction of $30 million annually in obesity costs, the research is not yet available to make that kind of forecast. But the preliminary results from a four-year USDA-funded research grant to determine the impact of CWK do look encouraging. The study has found that children enjoy cooking, whether it is in the classroom or at home. While such a conclusion might not sound terribly profound, it's certainly a principal assumption that every parent and teacher must learn to make. Confidence in cooking abilities, what educators like to call "self-efficacy," also increased significantly for children participating in CWK compared to children in nonparticipating schools. As we learned from Austin, self-confidence is a critical wall that everyone must climb. As might be expected, early research results found that preferences for fruits and vegetables were greater in children from CWK schools. And in what might be considered an "Aha!" moment for educators, nearly 99 percent of classroom teachers whose children participated in CWK said that it strengthened their students' learning in other curricula areas such as language arts and math.

Walters thinks that CWK works because food and the experience of food are at the heart of the program. "One little girl said to me after eating a fresh tomato, 'There is joy in my mouth.'" She believes that adults take food too seriously and have a tendency to get too pedantic about it. We know that telling children they have to eat their veggies because they are good for them doesn't work, but Walters also thinks that adults make food too cute. "We underestimate children's innate intelligence as well as their ability to choose healthy food and to not eat too much. We need to make food fun, which means encouraging children to be engaged with their food in a very direct and experiential way." An engaged child is actively absorbing knowledge and processing it. That is because they are in a stage of development where, as Jean Piaget, the father of childhood development theory, noted, they need concrete experience. If their hands are not in the soil planting a seedling, or not chopping a tomato for salsa that they will soon consume, their learning is truncated and the impact of the lesson diminished.

Walters has been a food educator for fifteen years. She is no less passionate about her work today than she was twelve years ago when I first met her. She notes that forty states have purchased CWK's curriculum, certainly a testament to the respect that others have for her work as well as to the soundness of her program's method. Her willingness to subject herself and her staff to the rigors and demands of a four-year government evaluation further suggests that Walters is hungry (and hopeful) to prove that CWK is an important part of the answer to food problems that are eating our young people alive. If the research project's preliminary data holds up through the final analysis, it will strongly suggest that every school district in America should adopt the CWK curriculum. At $90 a pop, it would be hard to imagine a better long-term investment in the health and well-being of our young people.

CHAPTER 9

GETTING OUR HEADS ABOVE THE PLATE

Primary and secondary schools offer us appropriate ground for planting and nurturing seeds in the fertile minds of young people. When this is done with care and consistency over time, it is reasonable for our communities to expect a sustainable yield of young people competently educated in food issues and capable of ensuring, at a minimum, their own dietary health. Can and should we expect more? Could we in fact hope for high school graduates who are able to understand the tensions between the alternative and industrial food systems, and what their roles as both consumer and citizen are? While I have met my share of precocious high schoolers who are well on their way to "getting it," what I have seen taking place in our nation's colleges and universities suggests that the makings of a food revolution may be under way. In the same way that America's campuses eventually brought the Vietnam War to a grinding halt forty years ago, today's students may be the grit that finally busts the gears of the industrial food machine.

Returning to your alma mater after an absence of thirty-six years is risky business. For one like myself, who was caught up in the raging conflicts of the day—Vietnam, civil rights, feminism, and environmentalism (not to mention sex and drugs and rock 'n' roll)—a visit to the old college campus can feel more like a veteran's return to Omaha Beach than a pleasant stroll down memory lane.

But ever the nurturing mother, Bates College in Lewiston, Maine, reached out to me. Not so much, I think, to heal old wounds (I doubt if the college registrar's office had accurately catalogued those), but because I had written a book about food and, perhaps more importantly, had devoted my professional life to promoting the cause of food justice. I was invited to spend a couple of days on campus—give a lecture, meet with classes, and hang out with students—to explore the unattractive underbelly of the American food system, in which hunger, food deserts, and obesity reign supreme.

This invitation was made possible by one of those events that most small-college development offices only dream about: an anonymous alumnus gift of $5 million. For a place like Bates, whose alums are significantly underrepresented among the ranks of the Fortune 500, and perhaps disproportionately present in the teaching and social work professions, a gift of this magnitude from a former student was probably celebrated with an all-night "kegger" at the president's house. But to top it off, the extraordinary donation was designated for, of all things, food! For Bates, this meant that the college would further a commitment it had made over ten years before to promote local and sustainable dining. Half of the money would be used to finish the campus's spanking new, state-of-the-art dining hall and to purchase local and organic food, and half would be used to undertake a yearlong discourse labeled Bates Contemplates Food. As Bates's president Elaine Tuttle Hansen put it, "We want to add to the understanding and knowledge about food on campus, about where our food comes from, and about the larger food system in which Bates is embedded. We don't want to forget . . . the big problems associated with the food system—from our dependence on petroleum and corn to diet-related diseases . . . to global hunger."

It was under these auspices that I gladly accepted the invitation, but not without reservations about the notion of "contemplating food." That smacked a bit too much of the kind of navel-gazing often associated with academia. As a campus antiwar activist, I was always frustrated, for instance, with the college's propensity to study peace rather than to vigorously oppose the Vietnam War. I eventually warmed to the task at hand, however, as I recalled that Bates had led the way many years back with local and sustainable dining, earning a national reputation as a leader in that fast-growing subculture of great campus eating experiences. I decided there's nothing academic about good food, locally sourced.

There was one more thing that made me eager for the engagement. I'm referring, of course, to that little incident reported in a *New York Times* story on college food in the spring of 2007. A college-shopping high school student had remarked that Bowdoin College's dining service food was superior to Bates's. Not only was Bates Contemplates Food an opportunity to even the score with the college's archrival—food having replaced football among many institutions of higher learning as the hallmark of a college's reputation—the initiative would raise the college food bar so high that all future pretenders would need grappling hooks to reach Bates's heights. I can be contemplative, but I can also be competitive.

My first engagement on campus was a career briefing for students who were interested in community food activism. Any doubt I might have had about the value of my visit was immediately emulsified by the dozen pairs of eyes turned earnestly in my direction. We discussed the roles of food activism, advocacy, and social justice in today's society. We talked about what it means to be an agent for change when powerful forces such as the industrial food system stand foursquare against such change. As a living and breathing testament to the fact that you can actually earn a living as a social activist (and even put your children through colleges comparable to Bates), I assured my attentive listeners that there were a growing number of jobs and career paths open to those who were interested in food activism—from seed to fork, from empowering the hungry to changing public policy.

Their interest in food work has been stimulated in part by the various community service opportunities that exist in Lewiston—many of which are supported by the college. As a former shoe and textile mill town down on its luck, the community offered a rich laboratory of experience for any student with a budding interest in social change. As of this writing, Lucy Neely (class of '09) and Kyra Williams ('09) are performing their AmeriCorps assignments with nonprofit food organizations in the West; Dani Scherer ('11) is managing the Lewiston Farmers' Market; and Molly Mylius ('11) started a campus herb garden adjoining the Dining Commons. Several other students are pursuing writing and research projects that address food issues. If the end result of contemplation is action, Bates appears to be increasing the number of students and graduates who want to engage both their heads and their hands in pursuit of justice and sustainability.

My next stop was the new Dining Commons, which I toured with Christine Schwartz, dining services director. I was as impressed with the amazing array of diverse foods as I was with Christine's rapport with her staff. Everywhere she went, Christine left a trail of smiles and good cheer in her wake. Everyone I spoke to was proud of his or her work and happy to talk about it. The students said dining service staff was accessible and always willing to listen to student feedback. The "napkin board" at the front of the hall was a combination gripe site and suggestion box where students registered their complaints as well as ideas for new dishes. But after eating a delicious lunch of Asian noodles, some local cheeses, and a Maine apple crisp, it was hard to imagine that there could ever be anything to quibble over. I guess that's what happens when your food expectations were shaped by the 1969 Bates Meal Plan ("Would you like the tube steak or the steak in a tube?").

As far as how the food is sourced, 30 percent of it is locally produced, including Maine-grown apples, pears, tomatoes, lettuce, potatoes, melons, and beef. This percentage puts Bates well out in front of the national college pack. By comparison, the 333 colleges that have signed onto the Real Food Challenge as of 2008 set a goal of 20 percent of their total food purchases that will be "local, environmentally friendly, socially just, and humanely raised" by 2020.

Target figures like these can be useful benchmarks to measure one kind of progress. They may even instill a healthy competition among colleges and universities. But what I find more telling is what those numbers say about the relationship between a college and its immediate community and region. Buying locally produced food is good for the local economy, reduces food miles (the carbon footprint), and puts students in touch with where their food comes from. Yes, that's all true. But as our sense of human intimacy and trust erodes in direct proportion to the expanding scale and complexity of the global food system, won't relationships that foster connections between a variety of community stakeholders become more valuable over time?

Christine points out that developing trust between Bates and Maine farmers is the key to offering ever-greater percentages of locally produced food. But it might also be the key to achieving more holistic relationships between the college and the Maine community. We see this developing now between other institutions across the country—public schools, colleges, hospitals—and their respective farms and farmland. This was certainly the case in Cleveland where, as we saw, City Fresh had developed a series of synergistic relationships between producers, the Cleveland Clinic, Oberlin College, and Case Western Reserve University. Consider the depth and breadth of these immediate food and farm connections, and estimate what they might yield in terms of spiritual, educational, and environmental returns. A local alliance of farmers and eaters, linked through a network of collaborative and mutually beneficial effort, suggests a higher quality of community life that we are now only beginning to sample. College food purchasing power is not just a regional economic engine; it may also serve as one of many building blocks in a more intimate form of community, one founded on both economic and social relationships. And if all of this sounds a bit utopian, or, more precisely, like we're rushing headlong into the past, think again. While this vision of the future may have its Waltonesque elements (that's Walton as in

John Boy, not Sam), our advancements in technology and distribution business models that support sustainable regional food systems may now equip us to avoid the limitations of the past.

But riding above whatever ideal notions we have of our food system is the undeniable popularity of sustainable and local eating across the college dining landscape. According to nationwide surveys of college students reported by the California Alliance with Family Farmers, students report that it is important that their college provide sustainably produced food (62 percent), and that the meat served was humanely raised (78 percent). Similarly, campus and student engagement in everything from community food banks to local farming is at an all-time high, as are the number of course offerings that address some aspect of the food system.

Food is everywhere on campus these days, not just in the cafeteria. As one who earned his community food system stripes running a breakfast program for low-income kids and organizing a food co-op during his years at Bates, I can remember feeling pretty lonely and not particularly cool. After putting in several hundred hours of community food work during my junior year (1971), I applied for independent study credit, a concept that was barely recognized at the time. Grudgingly, and only after being required to submit a lengthy paper, I was granted what amounted to half a course credit. My, times sure have changed!

Outside speakers on the topic of food and related subjects such as the environment are yet another feature of campus life. Food "rock stars" such as Michael Pollan and Bill McKibben are bringing "the word" to large audiences, extending the reach of their message far beyond a few courses and classrooms. Under the Bates Contemplates Food initiative, Michael Pollan not only filled the 900-seat college chapel to overflowing, but so many people were unable to gain admission that he had to give a second presentation.

Now it was my turn to speak at Bates, and though I did not manage to overflow the considerably smaller venue granted me, I did preach before two appreciative classes and one small hall filled with members of the Bates community. I told the assembled that we have two food systems in the United States—one for the poor and one for everyone else. Hunger, food insecurity, food banks, food stamps, and Wal-Mart are on the "menu" for those at the wrong end of the food gap, while local, organic, Whole Foods, farmers' markets, and community-supported agriculture farms (CSAs) are set graciously before those at the affluent end. The divide is wide, growing, and potentially disastrous for a nation that prides itself on its social equality and justice.

This message seemed to resonate with a respectable number of students. One graduating senior told me that while Bates is indeed a leader in improving an institution's relationship to food, it shouldn't "fall too heavily into self-congratulation when what justice demands of us is to ask ourselves what more we can do . . . and then do it." Another student noted that "coming to Bates and spending time in Lewiston [a working-class and economically struggling city] allowed me to fully understand that good local food is disproportionally something for the privileged. I think we should . . . bridge the gap between improving our dining services . . . while simultaneously reaching out to the local community to see how we can help each other."

A sophomore who had become particularly active both on and off campus in food issues felt that more hands-on learning opportunities should be provided to students. It wasn't enough, in her opinion, to talk about food problems—students should be able to apply their newfound knowledge immediately and directly. She said that "most of the dorms and houses don't have kitchens. . . . More cooking classes and interactive workshops would be wonderful."

This final remark made me wonder if perhaps it is time for the liberal arts to embrace the culinary arts. I can remember one semester of golf that I was required to take in order to complete my Bates-mandated physical education requirement. Given that the calories

I have burned from a lifetime of driving golf carts around the links are far fewer than the excess calories I've consumed from many years of ignorant food choices, a "phys-ed" cooking class would have served me far better.

I have learned over the course of thirty-five years of community food work that if you succeed in getting people's heads "above the plate," that is, they learn more about their food than simply how it tastes, you have accomplished something of importance. There can be little doubt that Bates Contemplates Food has done just that. Like anything else, however, this initiative has resonated more loudly with some students than with others. I have no doubt that the dedicated and avid group of foodies-in-training that I had the privilege to meet will make a profound contribution to changing the way America eats. For other students, who still regard food as only a source of fuel, I am confident that a year of college-level food talk can't help but leave an impression on their thinking. I'm also willing to predict that Christine Schwartz and her dedicated team will ascend to new heights of culinary excellence, that more farmers will enter the Bates food supply chain, that student gardens will sprout across campus, and that my little alma mater will stand at the head of a growing column of colleges and universities committed to walking the walk of a just and sustainable food system.

It is fascinating if not truly encouraging to watch the spread of food wisdom across hundreds and perhaps thousands of U.S. college campuses. While I can't compare the intensity of food activism today to the intensity of antiwar sentiment in 1970—death and the threat of death are powerful motivators—I can say that student awareness of the connection between food, health, and the environment runs deep and wide, and might just possibly land our food culture, if not our entire American culture, in a far better place than it is today. Some might question the role of higher education in preparing today's young people to become informed and effective food consumers and citizens. After all, the stated missions of most liberal arts colleges and the more technical or career-oriented paths available at larger universities don't suggest that they are preparing their students to take on the oligopolistic forces of multinational agribusiness. But imagine, just imagine, what effect millions of thoughtful and passionate young people leaving institutions of higher learning every year might have on our food system.

CHAPTER 10

FOOD SOVEREIGNTY
The Right to Control Our Food

A concept called food sovereignty entered the "foodie" vocabulary sometime in the last two decades. We're not sure when exactly, but we do know why: the phrase was born as the result of a threat.

Take away the ability to grow food, whether at an individual, community, tribal, or national level, and you can imagine the reaction it will provoke. Even when the force that is depriving you of your food assures you that plenty of other food will be available, history has demonstrated that such domineering types are not often true to their word. Yet through treaty agreements, colonization by settlers or food corporations, or the failure of national food systems, people have lost their right to grow food, and with that loss goes a precious set of associated skills and traditions, to say nothing of food security. And what stands out in these cases is a certain benign attitude on the part of the perpetrators, who truly believe that they are doing you a favor by relieving you of the onerous task of producing or at least managing your own food supply.

Though the right to produce one's own food is not enshrined in America's Bill of Rights, the growth of the industrial food system accompanied by the rise of nonagricultural lifestyles may one day provoke a campaign to seek such a constitutional amendment. Anyone who has had the chutzpah to actually turn his or her manicured front lawn into a large vegetable garden would no doubt encounter the scorn of neighbors to say nothing of the wrath of town planners. In only the last few years several cities—Cleveland,

Chicago, and San Francisco among them—have had to pass ordinances to allow homeowners to keep chickens and bees (yes, restrictions do apply). While the right to garden is not yet well formulated as public policy, local jurisdictions that do not make land available for community gardens, either deliberately or simply out of bureaucratic inertia, are de facto depriving "landless" citizens of the right to grow food. Similarly, the right to maintain a modicum of regional food security is undercut by the countless and often "under the radar" actions of states and localities that sacrifice farmland to development, foster conditions that are unfriendly to long-standing farm operations, or simply negate the importance of agriculture as an economic activity. And all of these actions and inactions are bolstered by the seeming abundance of the industrial food system which, like the "mocking self" in this book's opening parable suggests, has robbed us of the human imperative to produce our own food.

In many countries across the planet, movements have risen up to protect national food sovereignty and indigenous agricultural knowledge from both internal and external threats. In some ways those movements share a common seed stock with those that have promoted food self-reliance in the United States since the 1960s. But food sovereignty has a taproot that penetrates far deeper than the urge to achieve some measure of independence from the industrial food system. Food sovereignty in fact expresses a core human fear that if you are cut off from your most elemental sources of sustenance—the ones that derive from your unique soil, climate, and growing conditions—you have simultaneously severed a sacred bond with your culture, with your ancestors, and with Mother Earth. This commitment to preserving the actual as well as the potential ability to grow food applies as much to the individual backyard gardener as it does to a region wishing to protect and utilize its existing farmland, water, and other food-producing resources.

Native Americans may have been the first to lose food sovereignty, at least in more modern times in North America. From the white settlers' virtual annihilation of the buffalo to the forced placement of tribes on reservations, one tribe after another was deprived of its traditional food sources and relegated to eating "white man's food" in the form of donated agricultural commodities sold at overpriced trading posts. It was not only their natural food sources that were lost, but also the underlying basis for sacred traditions that centered on the harvest and the hunt. In effect, they were deprived of their reason for being (a kind of illegal seizure of the soul), and they succumbed to mental depression as well as the ravages of diabetes, which in some tribal communities affects 60 percent of the adults.

But like a war cry echoing across the plains, the call for food sovereignty has emerged in Indian Country as a way for Native Americans to take back their peoples' health and nature's sacred testament. In Okmulgee, Oklahoma, the Myskoke tribe's Food Sovereignty Initiative is working with tribal members to increase their food self-reliance with the sustainable production of both native and healthy nonnative crops. The goal is to improve the overall health of the community and to develop new economic opportunities focused on food and agriculture.

Like continental Native Americans, native Hawaiians were once 100 percent self-sufficient and regarded their coastal seas and island lands as their perpetual providers. But the white colonizers with their pineapple and sugarcane plantations saw it differently. Land that once grew traditional crops like taro became the province of corporate farms, and the native people themselves used agricultural wages to buy food imported from the mainland. But like other First People of North America, Hawaiian communities and organizations have been rallying across the state to restore traditional food, agriculture, and their respective traditions. One example is MA'O Organic Farms (MA'O being a Hawaiian acronym for "youth food garden"), which is focused on the mission of bringing food self-reliance to the Leeward coast of O'ahu Island. To this end it is developing youth leaders "who work within interdependent arenas of agriculture, economics, Hawaiian cultural practices, nutrition, and food sovereignty." With assistance from the Trust for Public Land, MA'O Farms successfully completed the acquisition of an eleven-acre farm property to use as a permanent home for its organic farming operations.

THE JICARILLA APACHE TRIBE—THE PAST MEETS THE FUTURE

Three buffalo cows and one bull stand in a small pen behind the Jicarilla Apache Cultural Center in Dulce, New Mexico. They are distant relatives of the vast herds that the Jicarilla tribe once hunted across a region that stretches from what is now Denver to the Texas Panhandle. As the only buffalo currently on the tribe's 870,000-acre reservation in western Rio Arriba County, these four critters may seem but a faint flicker of their ancestors' former glory. But as a reminder of the Jicarilla people's commitment to self-reliance and tradition, they stand as powerful symbols of a past that is now pointing the way to the future.

Bryan Vigil, one of the tribe's 3,200 members, stands at the center of an effort to restore the buffalo's prominence to the lives of his people as a source of food and cultural identity. "Buffalo means a lot to our Tribe," says Bryan. "Its meat is precious to our lives; the hides provide warmth and shelter; the tails are used as ceremonial rattles, and their beards are mixed with tobacco to smoke as a cure for headaches." The Jicarilla are exploring the restoration of buffalo on a larger scale, though it may be some time before they make a significant contribution to the tribe's food supply. But to move the process along, Bryan arranged a donation of sixty buffalo by the Colorado chapter of the Nature Conservancy. These were sold for $200 each to members of the tribe. One of Bryan's hopes for the restoration of buffalo is that it will lead his people back to more traditional diets—plants as well as native game—which will help reduce the incidence of diabetes.

In the meantime, Bryan is using the buffalo to reconnect the tribe's members, especially the young people, to their traditions. To this end, he leads youth groups on "survival camps," which are outdoor excursions that include identifying and using wild plants, starting campfires by rubbing two sticks together, sleeping in tee-pees, and, of course, eating buffalo.

Jesse Lefevre has worked closely with Bryan. As the Jicarilla Nation's head agent from New Mexico State University's Cooperative Extension Service, he typically puts in seventy hours each week to promote sustainable agriculture, rangeland education, livestock management, and youth programs. It is in this latter capacity that Jesse joins Bryan in his survival camps, and while not a Native American himself, he has worked with the tribe for fourteen years with its consent, collaboration, and respect. The young people look up to him, not only because he is a good six feet, three inches tall, but because they and other members of the tribe have learned that his intentions are good, an essential requirement for an "outsider" to gain trust from Native American groups.

The trust he has earned allows Jesse to work effectively with the tribe's 117 ranchers, who run 5,000 head of cattle across the tribe's rangeland. He has convinced them to reduce their herd size in order to improve the quality of the grazed grasses. Through Jesse's knowledge of federal programs, he has also been able to secure $2 million over the last few years from the USDA to make additional range improvements. And when the federal government's "one-size-fits-all" approach to making grants doesn't fit the practices and traditions of Indian Country (e.g., the federal government likes fences because they define ownership of property, but the Jicarilla don't believe in using them because their "property" is held in common), Jesse has shown remarkable creativity in "finessing" the system so that it works for everybody.

As all people know, food and economic self-reliance won't be achieved solely by employing the practices of the past or even by making wise use of natural resources. That is why Diana Pierce incorporates the past into the operation of a modern supermarket that harnesses the tribal members' buying power. Since 1988, Diana had managed an old, outdated food and general merchandise store in Dulce that had such a limited selection of items that most people had to make a two-hour round-trip drive to Farmington, New Mexico, or Pagosa Springs, Colorado, to do their major food shopping. Economists call this "leakage": money that could have stayed in the community to help its members was going elsewhere, where it did little good for the Jicarilla people. Since the small store also couldn't carry an adequate inventory of fresh produce and low-sugar products, it could do little to stem the rising tide of diabetes.

With the tribe's blessing and financial support (the Jicarilla are fortunate in that they control substantial oil and gas leases that produce ample revenue), Diana launched the development of a new, state-of-the-art 38,000-square-foot supermarket. She broke ground in August 2002 and held the store's grand opening in July 2003. The store is a jewel of supermarket design, both inside and out. Spacious, bright, and spanking clean, the store features murals that display spectacular mountain vistas and Apache legends. A mouth-watering produce department, shelf space enough for a full range of products, a top-of-the-line meat case, and take-out and prepared food vendors line three sides of the store. Add to this ample community meeting space and a huge back room replete with seven walk-in coolers and freezers, and it is clear that the Jicarilla Apache Supermarket would be the apple of any store manager's eye.

In only a little over a year the new store tripled the sales of the former one. It is a meeting place for the community and provides fifty full- and part-time jobs. Not only has the food-buying leakage stopped, but now shoppers come from around the region to shop in Dulce.

Through food-related economic development, careful use of its natural resources, and a respect for traditional practices, the Jicarilla Apache Nation is bringing self-reliance and health back to its people.

RUSSIA: GROW YOUR OWN OR DIE

In a country that has seen more than its share of social, economic, and political upheaval, the Russian people have proven surprisingly resilient in the face of Soviet-era food shortages and a centrally planned agricultural economy that often fell short of its production quotas. Images of Russians standing in line at state food stores and old women in babushkas selling unappetizing vegetables on street corners have always caused me to wonder how Russians manage to get by.

Unknown to most of us in the West, Russians have cultivated a large, vibrant gardening culture that, according to Leonid Sharashkin of the University of Missouri, represents 2.3 percent of the nation's GDP and is worth $14 billion annually. Fully 35 million Russian households, or 66 percent of the population, garden on what constitutes only 6 percent of the country's total agricultural land. But on this small proportion, located in public spaces and country dachas, family gardens that average less than one-quarter of an acre in size are producing 92 percent of Russia's potatoes, 77 percent of its vegetables, 87 percent of its berries and fruits, and a majority of its milk and meat. In other words, it is likely that Russians would not survive without this source of food, or if they were forced to rely on the country's industrial-sized farms for their basic needs.

While the Russians' unique form of food sovereignty does not appear to be under threat at this time, neither does it receive the amount of respect it deserves from official sources. Since this indigenous form of food production is not institutionalized within the more formal economic structure of Russia's national food system, tacit acceptance places it in a vulnerable position, especially in light of the vagaries of Russian politics. But what if (one could only hope) two-thirds of American households ripped up their lawns and started producing a percentage of food equal to the Russians in their front and backyards, community garden plots, country homes, and private golf courses? How would the industrial food system—supermarket chains, the oil industry, lawn-care companies, agro-tech firms—react to such a flagrant display of American individualism?

SOUTH KOREA AND U.S. FREE TRADE AGREEMENT: FORFEITING THE RIGHT TO GROW FOOD

The flight from Seoul to the Korean peninsula's southern coastline swept across Suncheon Bay. Spread below me and cradled by the surrounding mountain ranges was South Korea's rice bowl, a checkerboard pattern of yellow and tan paddies ripening in the October sun.

This was 2006, and at the same time that the rice farmers' small combines were separating the pods from their stalks, 350 South Korean and United States trade delegates were gathering less than 200 miles to the southwest on Jeju Island. The scene there was decidedly different from the idyllic one I witnessed from the air. Over 10,000 specially trained riot police were facing off against a nearly equal number of farmers who had come to protest round four of the U.S./South Korea bilateral free trade agreement (FTA) negotiations. What was at stake for these embattled forces? For U.S. and Korean business interests, it was billions of dollars in new markets for textiles, electronics, cars, movies, and agricultural goods. For the farmers, it was their livelihoods, Suncheon's rice fields, and South Korea's food sovereignty.

With the aid of my guide and translator, Dr. Chu, I toured the rice-growing area near Suncheon. I wanted to talk to a rice farmer and managed to persuade Dr. Chu to stop along the country road as soon as we spotted one. Unluckily for me, that farmer turned out to be Choi Chan-Sick, a sixty-six-year-old rice farmer who was fastidiously raking a six-foot-wide strip of rice that he and his wife were drying in the blacktop's breakdown lane. His face was so wrinkled it looked like a contour map of the hilly terrain that we found ourselves in. As further testament to a lifetime bent in service to his rice paddy, his back was so permanently hunched that I felt a sympathetic jolt of pain shoot up my spine.

Smiling in that slightly idiotic way that Americans do when they find themselves in unfamiliar cultural situations, I asked him through Dr. Chu how the rice harvest was going that year. Instead of the usual noncommittal farmer shrug that I had become accustomed to from taciturn New England farmers and New Mexico cowboys, Mr. Chan-Sick let forth such an angry blast of invective that both Chu and I braced ourselves for an impending attack from the five-feet-tall Korean. The angry farmer's words were accompanied by an equally furious waving of his arms that helped to propel the heated volley from his mouth, and forced me to move my head several times to avoid being struck by his whirling fists. From this tirade, which lasted several minutes, the only phrases I could discern were "United States" and "FTA." Unknowingly, as Dr. Chu would later explain, deleting most of the expletives for my benefit, I had walked into a passionate display of South Korean food sovereignty. And as the unfortunate representative of the United States at that time and place, I now felt like an ugly American.

Mr. Chan-Sick was referring to the free trade talks between the U.S, the world's largest economy, and South Korea, the world's tenth largest. Both countries were under immense pressure to fully open their markets, primarily for the benefit of South Korea's electronic cartels and U.S. automotive and agricultural corporations. Given that South Korea is the United States' seventh-largest trading partner—the two countries currently do $72 billion in business together—the stakes were extraordinarily high for both sides. But the sticking point in these negotiations was agriculture, the sector that tends to generate the most passion in trade talks worldwide. And with South Korea, the spanner came from both sides of the Pacific—Korean rice and American beef.

The centrality of farming to global trade became readily apparent to me while in South Korea. I had been invited to speak to local officials and farmers about the development of farmers' markets, food policy councils, and other direct farmer-to-consumer marketing strategies. My Korean hosts were not looking for better sources of organic arugula or marketing tips for kimchi. On the contrary, they were deathly afraid that the FTA would unleash a torrent of cheap American farm goods into their domestic markets and thereby destroy their indigenous agriculture.

While in Seoul, the nation's capital, I witnessed angry street demonstrations protesting the FTA with banners that portrayed Uncle Sam making Koreans slaves to American rice and beef. I heard Kim Jae-Im, the leader of a Korean women's farmer organization, shout in defiance at a rally, "We don't have to take American agricultural products!"

In a more sedate setting I talked with Dr. Ki-woong Lee, chairman of the Agriculture Economic Department at Suncheon National University. He told me, "Agriculture is the foundation of the Korean nation; it is a divine calling. Rice, especially, enjoys a near-mythical status and is eaten three times a day by most Korean households." With the possible exception of the Thanksgiving turkey, you couldn't find a food item in the United States that is as fused to our national identity as rice is to Korea's.

The massive scale of U.S. rice farms dwarfs the average 3.5-acre Korean farm, and of course so does the size and efficiency of U.S. production. Dr. Ki-woong Lee said that an open market for U.S. rice will cut the cost to Korea's consumers in half but would be the death knell for between 70,000 and 140,000 Korean farmers. "We've opened up over 4 percent of our rice market to foreign producers under the minimum market access quota established by the World Trade Organization," said Lee, referring to concessions South Korea made at earlier global trade talks. "But Korean rice farmers will never be able to compete with the U.S in the open market." As an economist who also consults regularly with the government, he went on to predict that an FTA will fail "if it means rice will lose."

The Korean debate over trade, rice, and the protection of food traditions was conducted with an intensity that I had never experienced anywhere else, even in the rarified food environment that saturates my hometown of Santa Fe. Both the near-violent out-bursts of farmers and the more reflective words of academics pro-vided a context, though admittedly a sad one, for the Korean farmer and martyr Lee Kyung Hae, who committed suicide at the world trade talks in Cancun, Mexico, in September 2003. Mr. Hae's ulti-mate act of protest was directed at the world's largest financial and national institutions, which were blind to the centrality of land, food, and culture in the lives of everyday people.

In Korea, hundreds of small rice paddies are tucked neatly into nearly every valley. Since 70 percent of Korea is mountainous, the farmers put virtually every uninhabited square foot of level ground into food production. Food is rarely treated as only fuel for the body but more as an opportunity for the celebration of family and community, something I observed at nearly every meal I ate in Korea. No matter how mundane the occasion, lovely silver bowls of rice, kimchi (pickled cabbage), and pork were passed and shared, with the younger eaters first serving the older ones, in ac-cordance with an age-old protocol.

In the same way that Korean eaters honor their social and cul-tural relationship to food, farmers recognize a sacred tie to their land. My colleague and traveling companion, Wayne Roberts, the director of the Toronto Food Policy Council, related a decidedly more pleasant encounter with a Korean farmer than the one I had. He told me about She-ik Oh, a peasant farmer outside of Seoul who was incorrectly introduced to Wayne by his translator as a "farmer." Bowing and smiling with consummate grace, Mr. Oh gently chas-tised the translator: "I am a peasant, not a farmer. Farmers work for money; peasants work because they love the land and are tied to it."

We would be unlikely to hear such soulful utterances from the likes of the American Farm Bureau, one of the agricultural organi-zations hungrily eyeing Korean markets. In response to South Ko-rea's stated reluctance to make rice a part of the multibillion-dollar negotiation, a Farm Bureau spokesman said, "Obviously, that's not going to work for us." And in a classic piece of patronizing American rhetoric, Alexander Vershbow, U.S. ambassador to South Korea at the time of the FTA talks, offered Koreans this sop for sacrificing their farmers on the altar of free trade: "As a result of the FTA, Koreans will enjoy lower food prices. . . . Money saved on food can be invested in education, leisure, and cutting-edge IT services—exactly the type of sectors that need to grow to provide future generations with well-paying jobs." Could one find a better twenty-first-century restatement of the Grand Inquisitor's major thesis? Of course, the good ambassador failed to mention that South Korea already has a vibrant economy, less poverty than the U.S., and one of the best-educated workforces in Asia.

Clearly, what's behind the U.S. government's noble impulse to free Koreans from the burden of growing their own food is America's industrial agriculture sector. Since U.S. farm production is growing at twice the rate of domestic consumption, agriculture is increasingly dependent on exports to survive. In fact, the U.S. now ships 30 percent of its total production out of the country— over $62 billion a year (2006 figures).

One cause of overproduction—hence the need to force U.S.-produced food down the throats of other nations—are federal crop subsidies that encourage unnecessary surpluses and unfairly enhance U.S. competitiveness in world markets. U.S. rice farms alone received $9.9 billion in crop subsidies from 1995 to 2004. The single biggest individual recipients from *all* federal agricultural programs during this period were three rice farmer cooperatives that took home nearly $1 billion in taxpayer largesse. In light of these numbers, it takes a special kind of moxie to demand that Koreans forsake their rice production to absorb America's publicly financed farm operations.

There are, of course, many well-reasoned arguments for eliminating tariffs and promoting open markets on a global scale. A vibrant exchange of goods between nations facilitates cultural exchange, a more cosmopolitan worldview, and even world peace (one representative of America's Farm Bureau who was part of an Asian trade mission told me in all seriousness that there had never been a war fought between two countries that both had McDonald's restaurants). And there are certainly good reasons to encourage trade in food as well (among them being my refusal to give up European cheeses).

But the ultimate economic rationale for accepting another nation's goods and no longer protecting your own is based on the principle of comparable advantage. Stated simply, countries that can produce, ship, and sell (for whatever reasons) a product of comparable quality cheaper than other countries will have the advantage in the marketplace. Lower Asian labor costs are why most of our clothing now comes from China. Rice farms of thousands of acres in Arkansas and California (having favorable rice-growing climates), supported by large federal subsidies and fueled by agro-industrial technology, are the reasons why we can sell lower-cost rice to the Koreans.

But when it comes to the negotiation of trade agreements, comparable advantage is the only concept on the table. For Korea, as well as many other nations, the principles of food sovereignty and food security are just as important as the economics. Food sovereignty addresses the right of all nations to make their own food policies in order to feed their people because food is central to human and national survival. That right cannot be trumped solely by market forces.

With respect to food security, Korea has suffered as much war, starvation, and economic hardship as any nation in the twentieth century. Why, then, should it relinquish rice production, its most important crop, to the U.S? Should American farms stop producing beef because Australians can do it cheaper? Should we plow under our apple orchards because Chinese apple-farming costs are lower? With our food system as dependent on declining energy resources as it is, a rational approach to food security suggests that food supply lines should be shortened and localized, not lengthened and globalized. And when food and farming are so finely woven into the fabric of a nation's history and culture, why should they become pawns on a chessboard dominated by other major industrial sectors like autos, electronics, and textiles?

We could easily dismiss the issue of free trade as one that is too distant from our daily lives to matter. But when free trade crosses into the principle of food sovereignty, it forces us to confront that adage that what's good for the goose is good for the gander. If we think that South Korea should remove its tariff barriers to allow the import of cheaper U.S. rice, then shouldn't the U.S. remove tariff barriers to the import of agricultural goods from any other country? Cheaper apples from China may mean that the lovely orchards of upstate New York are turned into housing lots. Cheaper soybeans from Brazil may mean the end of the vast stretches of soybean fields across the Midwest. Cheaper tomatoes from Mexico may mean the end to Florida's winter tomato crop. The need for other countries to determine what's best for their farmers, food security, and significant cultural practices must be respected and cannot be overridden by the bottom-line forces of the industrial food system.

To close the story, for now, on the Republic of Korea–United States Free Trade Agreement, the treaty was signed by both countries' presidents on June 30, 2007. As Dr. Ki-woong Lee predicted, rice was forced off the table by the South Koreans, who essentially told the U.S. that no treaty could be completed if it was forced to remove its rice tariffs. The U.S., however, extracted other agricultural concessions from South Korea, which must reduce its 40 percent tariff on U.S. beef imports over fifteen years, and allow $1 billion worth of other U.S agricultural imports. At the moment, beef remains an obstacle to the treaty's approval by the U.S. Senate since South Korea has imposed a health ban on the import of U.S. beef since BSE ("mad cow disease") was discovered in U.S. cows. Of course, this action has provoked strong outrage from the U.S. cattle industry, which has been more than matched by strong and sometimes violent protests by South Koreans who do not want the U.S. to impose its beef on them.

Finally, the agreement allows other farm exports to South Korea to become duty free immediately. And in order to protect and diversify its agricultural sector, South Korea will invest $119 billion in aid to South Korea farmers over the next ten years to offset the effects of the agreement.

As of this writing, neither the South Korean National Assembly nor the U.S. Congress has approved the treaty.

CHAPTER 11

FOOD CITIZENS, UNITE!

What has distinguished the alternative food movement more than anything else over the past ten years has been the meteoric growth in consumer food knowledge. Never have so many become so smart so fast about what they eat. Farmers' markets and Whole Foods would never have ascended so rapidly without the legions of eaters who now obsess daily over the impact of every bite on every molecule of their flesh. The informed food consumer is a formidable opponent to the industrial food system, indeed; but just as necessary, perhaps more so, is the informed food citizen. This is the person who sees the connection between the food he or she eats and the laws, budgets, and regulations that make up what is called public policy. Moreover, the wily and effective food citizen is the one who knows how to manipulate the levers of policy and political power to make the alternative food system more prevalent in the lives of millions, maybe even billions. Let's take a look at how the game is being played at the local and state levels of government.

The Albuquerque high school auditorium was nearly full. Onstage sat a dozen state officials and physicians and other health professionals, listening intently to a parade of parents, teachers, civic leaders, and even the occasional student—all speaking in favor of a proposal to ban sugary soft drinks and to require the state's public schools to offer healthier food.

Then it was the other side's turn. Standing in a carefully coifed cluster, immaculately attired and bristling with confidence, America's beverage industry representatives made their case for the retention of soda in New Mexico's public schools. Each of the speakers—none of whom were state residents—announced their names, punctuated with an alphabet soup of credentials that spanned the range of most known health disciplines. They argued that soft drinks are not as unhealthy as people think, that the real culprit in America's obesity crisis isn't too many calories but too little exercise, and that it is simply not right to deprive schoolchildren of the nation's iconic soda brands.

These arguments were as disingenuous as the case for healthy school food was compelling. But public institutions aren't always rational, nor do they change easily, and no matter how "right" your arguments are, corporations don't give up millions of dollars without a fight. A backroom deal between state officials and the beverage industry nearly scuttled the proposed reforms. But the light of day was too bright, and the voice of citizens too strong. Today, the cafeterias of New Mexico's public schools no longer sell Pepsi or Coke. In their place, students find 100 percent fruit juice, water, and locally produced apples, green chile, and salad greens.

The victory was by no means inevitable. The state's nutrition reforms were the direct result of work done by the New Mexico Food and Agriculture Policy Council, an organized group of farmers, nutritionists, educators, activists, and others on a mission for healthier food.

Big decisions about food, nutrition, and agriculture used to be the purview of a small cadre of agribusiness corporations and political heavy hitters. But more and more, people are realizing that decisions that affect their food and health are too important to leave in the hands of others. Around the country citizens are organizing food policy councils (FPCs) to hold their elected officials accountable for junk food in schools, food insecurity in poor neighborhoods, and the future of agriculture.

The FPC movement started more than twenty-five years ago in

Knoxville, Tennessee, and now includes about 100 councils across North America. The councils come in many shapes and sizes—some organized by citizens, some established formally by an ordinance, state statute, or executive order. And increasingly, these food policy councils are publicly asserting that the nation's food system must serve a triple bottom line—one that is good for producers, for the environment, and for all consumers, including low-income households.

FOOD DEMOCRACY AT WORK

Agitated chatter spilled out of the meeting room at the Boulder County Natural Resources building in Colorado. Over beer and pizza (both locally produced) the twelve members of the newly appointed Boulder County Food and Agriculture Policy Council were putting the finishing touches on a strategic plan to boost the county's production and distribution of local food.

The discussion grew tense when one member protested that her ideas and values were not reflected in the plan's current draft. Cindy Torres, the council chair, called a time-out. The issue wasn't about whether the member's perception was right or wrong, the question was how everyone's point of view could be accommodated in order to bring the group to consensus. Because local food systems are large and diverse, food policy councils are committed to listening to everyone's ideas. Indeed, the dissenting member had taken a position that so narrowly defined sustainable agriculture that most other forms of agriculture would be excluded from future council discussions. This would have been harmful to the principles of inclusivity and transparency that the Boulder folks were trying to uphold. But as discussion resumed, the reluctant member calmed down, put aside her doubts, and accepted compromise language that would give all sides a seat at the table. Time, patience, and a respect for everyone's opinion won the day.

"We want everyone to know they have a voice in our food system," says Torres. "Yes, we focus on environmental sustainability, but in order for our work to have a long-term impact, we must also work on social sustainability." Though inclusivity and consensus building inevitably take longer and sometimes wear people out, it's time well spent, in Torres's opinion. "At first we had only a collection of special interests. But now we have a vision that everyone can share and work for." With a smile, Torres adds that food policy councils are "like being in a big family. All those people aren't going away, so you better learn to deal with them."

The family metaphor is especially apt in light of the localized focus of food policy councils. The network of community relationships that binds people at a local level can often get messy. But it's that proximity—call it a kind of down-home frisson—that gives food policy councils their strength. At the federal level, where Congress and the administration make national food policies like the Farm Bill, the average citizen's voice gets lost. But when food policy councils confront a local school board or state legislature, elected officials must listen and work with them.

This strategy has been successful in New Mexico, where the council has worked with public and private partners to advocate successfully for increased state funding for farmers' markets and the federal- and state-funded Farmers Market Nutrition Program. It has also been successful in promoting state policies to preserve farmland, source more locally produced food for the public schools, and develop retail food stores in rural food deserts.

As we've seen, Connecticut's food policy council (which includes everyone from the state's Farm Bureau and grocery industry to organic farmers and food banks) made a long-term commitment to farmland preservation that has paid off in the form of significantly more state funding to purchase easements. More recently, the council has turned its attention to developing markets for locally produced food in public institutions like schools and prisons. According to their chairperson, Linda Drake, "The barriers to getting local foods in institutions can be enormous, but we now have several groups working together to figure out what we can do to eliminate those barriers." Developing new facilities for livestock slaughtering and meat processing in the New England region, where they have virtually disappeared, is one of the food policy council's highest priorities.

Food policy councils' commitment to building a "big tent," open to many interests, is starting to pay off in other communities as well. Cleveland's agencies and organizations, for example, have "brought together an amazing group of food system stakeholders who have a vision for a just and sustainable local food system," according to Jennifer Schofield, cofounder of the Cleveland–Cuyahoga County Food Policy Council. Like many so-called rust-belt cities, Cleveland has lost a staggering number of residents and supermarkets, leaving citizens stranded amid large tracts of vacant land with no place to shop. But Schofield saw vacant lots as future mini-farms, and the remaining corner stores as potential outlets for healthy food, not just candy, tobacco, and lottery tickets. "Anybody in their right mind knows that Cleveland's economic future isn't with the Fortune 500. We need to stimulate small, local businesses like food and gardening."

But how do you start up agriculture in the middle of a city, and on a scale that will make a difference? The food policy council tackled that question by seeking citywide policies that could open possibilities for urban farming. They found a champion in City Councilor Joe Cimperman, a ten-year veteran of Cleveland's Thirteenth Ward. As a disciple of the power of zoning to improve a community's quality of life, Cimperman has placed the city's zoning code at the service of local food advocates. "If city government was a faith," Cimperman proclaimed, "zoning would be its highest sacrament."

This strategy to employ all of the policy tools available to a city to the problems of food security and economic development has served as a perfect complement to the work of Maurice Small and City Fresh. As much by temperament as by personal passion, people like Maurice are not patient with the sometimes plodding ways of government. Like the iron tip at the head of the battering ram, they must use their mind and muscle to directly confront the challenges and opportunities before them. But without the bigger shoulders of government to add weight and momentum, the results will be limited and the overall impact marginal. When an entire city can get behind innovative work like that of City Fresh, minor miracles can become everyday occurrences.

Cimperman and the FPC have secured a zoning change that permits community gardening and the raising of chickens and bees (four hens, no roosters, and one hive per house lot). They are now working on new zoning to create larger plots of one acre or more for commercial-scale agriculture. Cleveland's economic development funds are being used to make micro-loans to urban farmers, and the city is studying how it can use its current food purchasing power to buy more locally produced food. "Urban farming can be transformative in terms of the economy, nutrition, health, and public safety," Cimperman says. "Our goal is to make Cleveland a national leader in the local food economy."

Similar approaches have succeeded in Portland, Oregon, where the fifteen-member City of Portland and County of Multnomah Food Policy Council has encouraged the city to open up more land for community gardens through their Diggable City project, which has turned the public spotlight on the need for more urban plots. Even though 3,000 people currently till the city's community gardens, there are still 1,000 gardener wannabes on a waiting list.

Portland is also thinking beyond garden plots as it attempts to seize control of its own food destiny. The council is working with the region's planning commission to encourage the inclusion of food access, affordable food, and the viability of state agriculture in the region's five-year comprehensive land use plan. Should it succeed, it will be the first time any major American city has recognized food and agriculture as key issues in city and regional planning.

In Missoula, Montana, the Community Food and Agriculture Coalition has taken new ground in the battle to preserve the Bitterroot Valley's historic farm and ranch communities. The coalition, which includes a wide variety of local food and farm interests, was successful in placing one of its staff members on a county land use commission that oversees planning and development. After working with the coalition to map the area's soils to identify those most suitable for agriculture, the land use commission adopted recommendations that require it to consider the impact of future subdivisions on existing farms and ranches. Since the coalition has a seat at the commission's table, it has been able to play a vital role in conserving prime agricultural land while steering development into less sensitive areas. This has been an innovative role for citizen groups like the coalition.

Getting local food systems to the table of municipal and county decision makers is often the result of a considerable amount of advance work and old-fashioned community organizing. According to Bonnie Buckingham, formerly with the Missoula food bank and cofounder of the coalition, it began with an extensive assessment of the community's food system. This involved looking into every nook and cranny of the region to determine where the producers were, where the people were who needed food, and where the gaps and failures in the food supply and distribution chain were. In other words, the group was searching for opportunities to improve life for both farmers and consumers.

What quickly became apparent was that many farm owners wanted their land to be preserved for farming—they didn't want to see the fields they had worked so hard and for so long sprouting McMansions. At the same time, consumers wanted reliable sources of locally produced food, and they would feel more secure if they could count on their own farmers to maintain their food supply. This sense of local food security was not a romantic notion dreamed up by a few rabid foodies; the assessment found both the need and the opportunity to make that food available to schools and food stamp recipients and other lower-income consumers. In effect, there was a strongly felt and widespread community need to close the gap between food's producers and consumers.

As Buckingham said, "It's easy to get your voice heard in Missoula, and it's easy to gain access to policy makers." That's true, and it's why groups like the Community Food and Agriculture Coalition have made great strides in realizing a comprehensive vision for the future of their region's food system. But not only are voices easier to hear at the local level, there are now more of them. It's safe to assume, for instance, that the issues Missoula has addressed recently would have been ignored only ten years ago. By way of example, an ordinance that came before the Missoula commissioners to permit backyard chicken raising—a maximum of six hens—drew hundreds of supportive people to a public hearing, a big enough flock to gain overwhelming support for the ordinance. Whether "legalizing" the growing of food and raising of food animals (who would ever have thought that such basic human activities might become illegal) or securing the future of nearby farms and farmland, citizens are finding their voices and using the levers of government to control their local food destinies.

Places like Missoula, Cleveland, Portland, Connecticut, and New Mexico have made important food policy gains. Not only are they revamping the way that they produce and distribute food, they are in some cases beating back the darker forces of the industrial food system. There is hope on the land and promise in the air that the decades of struggle for a just and sustainable food system are starting to pay dividends. But there is concern as well that it is only the low-hanging fruit being picked, and that much bigger and more consequential battles are looming on the horizon. So much is at stake and too much money is on the table for anyone to believe that the alternative food movement can rest on its laurels.

SHOOTOUT ON THE FRONT RANGE

With its sprawling farmers' market, wall-to-wall health food stores, and pure Rocky Mountain air, Boulder, Colorado, is nearly the last place on earth you'd expect to find a clash between the alternative and industrial food systems. Yet in spite of the soft scent of paradise wafting down its idyllic lanes, trouble came to town in the form of six farmers who had the gall to ask the county for permission to plant genetically modified sugar beet seed on publicly owned farmland. It was as if a bunch of rowdies had shown up at Fenway Park wearing Yankees caps; nothing could have been more anathema to the otherwise mellow folks of Boulder.

All ninety-eight seats in the Boulder County public hearing room were filled. The overflow crowd spilled into the hallway and down the stairs, where people listened to the proceedings through a public address system. The hearing, conducted by the Boulder County Food and Agriculture Policy Council, began at 5:30 p.m. and didn't conclude until fifteen minutes past midnight. The topic—whether to permit the planting of GMO sugar beets on farmland owned by the County of Boulder—would later be described by Cindy Domenico, a member of the board of county commissioners, as "the most complex, interesting and deep issue that has ever come up here since my time on the board."

Not only would it be one of the most powerful issues to come before a veteran body of elected officials, it would be the first issue to come before the still wet-behind-the-ears Food Policy Council, a one-year-old publicly appointed group whose ink wasn't even dry on its strategic plan. As the holder of 26,000 acres of cropland managed by the county's Parks and Open Space Department, the county commissioners had punted the ball to the council to hold a public hearing, gather information on one of most contentious issues facing food and farming today, and make its recommendation to the commissioners. The council's members may have been hungry for action, but they had been hoping for a few easy skirmishes first.

The county was in the unique position of deciding on the GMO request because it had the foresight over the course of many prior years to purchase substantial tracts of open land. The county had set the land aside to keep it from development, conserving it for open space, wildlife habitat, and crop production. In short, this was the people's land because public resources had been used to secure its protection and to serve the public interest in perpetuity. The farmland portions were leased to numerous farmers for what has traditionally been the production of large-scale commodity crops, including 1,500 acres that had been leased for GMO corn production several years ago. At the time that decision was made—over the concerns of many citizens and prior to the creation of the county FPC—it was stipulated that any future lease decisions involving GMO seed would have to be approved by the county as an entirely separate transaction. The time had come once again to confront the question, but this time the county commissioners had a food policy council to turn to.

Not only was the hall packed to the gills, the people were agitated, and many were carrying signs (all in opposition). You could say the air was redolent with the acrid sweat of democracy. In anticipation of a big and boisterous turnout, the county had assigned a security person, who was, as Cindy Torres would later put it, "a very big guy" (he did have to escort one particularly incensed opponent from the building). Torres called the meeting to order and reminded those who would testify that in order to accommodate everybody there would be a three-minute limit on comments. A total of fifty-eight citizens would be heard that night, and the scorecard would show that forty-seven of them expressed adamant opposition to the use of GMO seed on public land, while the rest offered only lukewarm support.

Depending on whose witnesses were being heard, the science and risk associated with GMOs was either irrefutably reassuring, murky, or downright horrifying. Proponents claimed that the biotechnology had been thoroughly tested and bore the USDA's goodhousekeeping seal of approval. Opponents argued that "seed drift" was inevitable and would contaminate non-GMO crops, thus rendering them unsalable in markets where genetically engineered food was unwelcome. Competing definitions of "sustainability," "farm viability," and "democracy" infused the debate. The six farmers requesting permission to use GMO sugar beet seed warned of dire consequences to their livelihoods and agriculture in general if their request was denied. One of them said, "Of the 1,100 acres [I currently farm on public land], 14 percent is sugar beets [currently conventional seed]. Those sugar beets contribute to 32 percent of my income. There just isn't another viable crop out there. . . . By removing Roundup Ready sugar beets, you have essentially delivered the death blow to another independent farmer."

As the clock struck midnight and the grueling hearing came to a close, the council members prepared to vote. All of them expressed sympathy for the farmers and the larger economic plight of agriculture. All of them acknowledged that this was public land and that the needs of the community's health and well-being were paramount. Some wondered why more organic and sustainable forms of agriculture, particularly ones that would produce food for local consumption, couldn't be encouraged on this land. And all of them shared their anguish and their feelings that this was a "no-win" situation. The vote was 9 against the use of GMOs and 3 in favor.

The Colorado Farm Bureau would later describe the action of the food policy council and the community's opposition thus: "Anti-agriculture activists in Boulder County have stepped up their efforts in the media to slander and malign sugar beet production on open space land. Activists are lining up to attack the Roundup Ready Sugar beets." The bureau characterized a film being shown in Denver called *The World According to Monsanto* as a "radical French-made documentary," and noted that someone who works for Transition Colorado, the organization sponsoring the film, was also a member of the Boulder food policy council. One individual referred sympathetically to the applicant growers as "small farmers [who] didn't stand a chance against big-city activists." Many people who disagreed with the council's decision noted that conventional sugar beet production, at least on the scale of thousands of acres and tilled with repeated passes of energy-intensive farm equipment, might even be less sustainable than the no-till/low-till form of agriculture allowed by using Roundup Ready seed.

Obviously the blaming and framing games had been well rehearsed in advance and were ready for prime time as soon as the council's vote was announced. Large commodity growers suddenly became "small" and "independent." Those who criticize corporate giants with ignoble track records are the "radical French." And citizens who responsibly spoke their mind in accordance with the democratic process are smeared as "big-city activists."

What was lost in the accusations and of course ignored by the agribusiness representatives was the fact that Boulder's growers had been forced into a box by Monsanto. The sugar beet producers submitted their request to use GMO seed because they were unable to purchase conventional seed. Two years ago 60 percent of the sugar beet seed on the market was GMO. Today it is 95 percent. Not only did Monsanto jam the farmers into a corner, it made it easy to brand the Boulder community as anti-farmer bogeymen hell-bent on putting poor, salt-of-the-earth farmers out of business. As one farmer at the hearing admonished the anti-GMO speakers, "I don't believe that anybody has the right to take the tool [of GMO seeds] away from the farmers." But it's Monsanto and other biotech firms that are taking tools away from farmers.

Council chairwoman Torres defended the process and its outcome: "Civic engagement is underutilized in our country and the movement that empowered so many to speak out recently in Boulder was not anti-farmer. It was anti-GMO. The farmers took the fall for the GMO industry." There are many failures and gaps represented by the shoot-out in Boulder, ones that the industrial food system is not genuinely interested in addressing. Industrial food interests create conflicts that attempt to present consumers as uninformed and unsympathetic to agriculture. They also tend to use the science selectively in their favor and to further marginalize educated laypeople who struggle to understand the complexities of biotechnology. According to Torres, who posted an extensive analysis of the events on the Huffington Post, she was called by a university professor from Colorado who advised her to be cautious in expressing anti-GMO sentiments "because of the biotech industry's policy of suppressing the opposition."

She would be far from the first person to be singled out for intimidation by the agriculture-industrial complex. Because of my and my family's own activism, we have received threatening or silent phone calls at 3:00 in the morning. On a larger stage, I have alluded earlier to the way that New Mexico's "Big Ag" players work to suppress research that may be critical of their activities; and on the state level opposition to legislation, even when it is benign to Big Ag's interests, can turn routine lobbying into a form of retribution. The tactics I described earlier that were used to oppose the expansion of workers' compensation coverage to agricultural workers were mild compared to others I have seen, which would be more worthy of Al Capone. In many states across America, Big Ag sometimes talks loudly and sometimes softly, but it always carries a big stick.

On August 25, 2009, the Boulder County Board of Commissioners wrapped up a seven-hour meeting "in front of hundreds of county residents" by voting to delay their final decision on GMO sugar beet seeds. The petition filed for GMO seed use was withdrawn by the farmers. The board said it wanted to see a comprehensive plan for the county's 26,000 acres of cropland that would include provisions for organic acreage, rules for herbicide use, and a commitment to maintaining the financial viability of family farms in the Boulder region. A further obstacle to widespread GMO use arose when a federal judge in San Francisco ruled on September 21, 2009 that the U.S. Department of Agriculture improperly allowed the commercialization of genetically modified sugar beets. Apparently, the USDA rushed through the approval process without preparing an environmental impact statement for the herbicide-tolerant plants. While the long-term implications of the ruling do not necessarily signal a death knell for GMO sugar beets, it should slow their further use. But at the very least, the federal court ruling provides several layers of vindication for the Boulder Food Policy Council.

We can expect the conflict to rage on between the assumed right of industrial agriculture to do whatever it wants whenever it wants, and the growing fears and doubts of consumers and communities. Not even in Boulder, with its strong alternative roots and gregarious organic culture, is there a resolution in sight or a reason for the pro–alternative food system advocates to rest easy. The GMO industry and its front men aren't going away. There will be well-financed and amply lawyered attempts by industrial agriculture to assert its claim that it is entitled to choose the direction of our food system without outside interference or consultation. But in the meantime, food citizen democracy appears to be a tentative winner, albeit battered and bruised. Though one member of the Boulder food policy council resigned in the aftermath of these events, apparently finding the kitchen a little too hot for her liking, the existence of an informed and committed group of members kept the beast at bay, at least for now, but more importantly, those members had the courage and the resolve to wade into the fray. Yes, democracy prevailed at the foot of the Rockies, but as Torres said, "I think we can all anticipate more conflicts arising between farmers and eaters because we are only now recognizing that consumers have a role in our food and farm industry. Together, the farmers and consumers must hold the industry accountable, otherwise they will do everything they can to divide us." As new voices speak out through councils and similar local organizations, there's hope that public policy will start delivering what people really need—healthy, affordable, sustainable food. Putting control back in the hands of the people is rough business. But so is democracy.

CHAPTER 12

REFLECTIONS ON FOOD DEMOCRACY
A Chat with Two Visionaries

With the growing recognition that every bite we take may have profound consequences for other humans and the environment, something as mundane as three meals a day takes on a highly elevated meaning. The invisible dinner companion—the place setting with no one at it—becomes our values, a combination of emotions and ideas that influence what we eat. We believe, for instance, in democracy, and the right of people to make their own decisions and to control their own destinies. We also value the concept of legacy—the wish to leave behind healthy children, a clean planet, and sustainable natural resources. When people talk about food, the primacy of values, to say nothing of the emotional chords that are struck when the subject arises, becomes obvious.

Food democracy. People power. Empowerment. Good food. These are phrases designed to stir our emotions, but more importantly change our behavior and move us to action. They help us dig a little deeper into ourselves in the fervent hope that we might find the will and the clarity of thought to take on something that is stronger than ourselves but, if left unchallenged, remains a palpable threat to the people and places we love.

Organizing all of this human energy toward some end, such as deep and transformational food system change, is both a talent and a calling. Helping others recognize that their values are shared by others, and then creating a structure that will enable them to turn those values into concrete action, is what organizers do. These people are necessary players among a cast of thousands who speak their lines from countless community stages that sometimes morph into national platforms. They are practical, multiskilled, strategic as well as tactical, and possessed of a fiery intellect that enables them to translate complex and competing analyses into terms and actions capable of changing communities. Call them thought leaders or servant leaders, they don't lead with their egos or the false blandishments of charisma; they effectively enable others to discover and express for themselves the beliefs that they've held all along.

To understand what this kind of leadership looks like, I spent some time with two leading organizers/social entrepreneurs, Richard Pirog and Brahm Ahmadi. Rich is the associate director of the Leopold Center, which is based at Iowa State University and is charged with conducting research and assisting the state's food and farm stakeholders to promote a sustainable food system. Brahm is the executive director of People's Grocery, a nonprofit organization that is attempting to develop the food self-reliance and wealth of the West Oakland community in California's Bay Area. Their geographic areas and food systems are as different as night and day—Iowa sprawls across 56,000 square miles, much of which is devoted to the production of hogs, corn, and soybeans, while West Oakland is barely 5 square miles and is a classic food desert with the exception of only a few urban gardens. But the resemblance between the two leaders' outlooks and organizations is uncanny.

Ironically, Rich Pirog looks at Iowa's mammoth agricultural sector as an underdeveloped resource that may serve the global economy tolerably well—Iowa is the nation's leading corn and ethanol producer—but has not come close to fulfilling its potential for feeding the state's citizens and meeting their nutritional needs. Iowa's official Web site touts itself as "the food capital of the world." Pirog would be happy if Iowa could become the food capital of Iowa. Based on a study conducted by the Leopold Center (which has churned out more research on local and sustainable food systems than just about any other academic institution), the existing agricultural economy, with its increasing emphasis on energy rather than food, may not be the best bet. If Iowans started eating five servings a day of fresh fruits and vegetables (the national average is currently closer to two), and all those servings came from Iowa producers, 4,100 new jobs would be created by this "eat and grow local" approach. But what Big Ag doesn't like to hear is that this healthy diet could be grown at 1/30th the cost of developing twenty-six ethanol plants and would require the conversion of only 34,000 acres of Iowa's existing cropland.

"It's those kinds of numbers that have economic development officials drooling," said Pirog. "Pottawattamie County [home to Council Bluffs, Iowa] is kicking in $30,000 per year for each of the next four years for local food and agriculture because they see it as a better economic engine than other options." Economic development is only one of the benefits of a locally oriented food system. The Leopold Center's "Five-a-Day" study decided not to quantify the health benefits because of methodological difficulties, but one would have to assume that there would be measurable improvements when a large segment of the population shifts its diet to more fruits and veggies. Healthier people, with reduced rates of obesity and diet-related illnesses like diabetes, result in lower health care costs for individuals, health insurance providers, and taxpayers.

Brahm Ahmadi has a similar view of his food economy, albeit from another angle. West Oakland has 30,000 people and fifty liquor stores, but hasn't had a supermarket in four years. People's Grocery was founded with the mission to address the huge health disparities and social injustices that exist in this predominantly African American community compared to the surrounding Bay Area. The organization has developed urban agriculture projects and pioneered an innovative mobile van delivery network that buys local food for distribution (in "Grub Boxes") to neighborhoods where grocery stores fear to tread. Though these projects have worked well, Ahmadi couldn't help but think that they weren't enough and that there were bigger fish to fry.

"I think about what Van Jones said, 'Many communities have been serviced into poverty,' and what places like West Oakland don't need are more social services, but more jobs, businesses, and wealth—wealth that people create and own." And like Pirog at the Leopold Center, Ahmadi went about looking at the food-buying potential of his community. "People think West Oakland has no wealth; look at it and you see a community that was cut to ribbons by the BART line and endless miles of highways: abandoned by heavy industry, which also robbed West Oakland of its middle class. But our market research found that residents buy $45 million of food every year. Nearly all that money leaves the community. Why can't we keep it here?" asked Ahmadi.

People's Grocery is recapturing a small percentage of that wealth through its gardening and delivery projects, but Ahmadi's hope is to develop a grocery store that can capture at least 30 percent of those food dollars now going elsewhere and, at the same time, create a couple of hundred new jobs. But the bigger target he's aiming at is community ownership in this and future enterprises. That would necessitate some kind of hybrid business model, one that crosses a well-managed and profitable supermarket with some form of community and worker ownership: not necessarily a majority share, mind you, but enough to begin to rebuild the wealth of West Oakland. "There's an imperative for greater economic control," said Ahmadi, "whereby people shift from being passive consumers to becoming active stakeholders."

But what is the path to a new food economy, one built on a foundation of local buying power and other food-related assets? After all, what is being proposed here requires not only sophisticated business acumen but a scale and type of social organizing and networking that has not been well tested in this country. Interestingly, Pirog from Iowa's sprawling prairie and Ahmadi from postindustrial Oakland envision similar road maps. They want to build multistakeholder and multicultural movements, develop indigenous leadership, and organize themselves around values of transparency, trust, and the transfer of knowledge.

"Of all the things I've done over the years," said Pirog, "I am proudest of graduating four MBAs from Iowa State who also minored in sustainable agriculture." These are the kind of new leaders that Pirog hopes to cultivate more of. They are the new renaissance men and women of food and farming who can plant one foot in the business world and one foot in the alternative food system world without becoming schizophrenic. He sees the need to create a new generation of professionals—from technical to teaching, from the community college to the graduate level. In an interesting twist on inclusivity, Pirog also thinks that more leaders from the food industry should be brought along into the alternative food movement, perhaps through academic mediums. He cites such highly rated corporate talent as Rick Schneiders, the retired CEO of the Sysco Corporation, one of the country's largest buyers of food for food service accounts. Under Schneiders's leadership, Sysco developed a number of initiatives across the country to increase the purchase of locally and sustainably produced food.

Where Pirog's thinking and work may make their greatest contribution is in their ability to strengthen regional food systems. In essence, he envisions and is beginning to develop local and regional networks in Iowa whose members' work is synchronized and additive, meaning that there is coordination, cooperation, and a continual process of building on one another's experience and knowledge. To visualize what that might look like, think of the opposite—the industrial food system sprawling across the globe in an uncoordinated and highly competitive fashion, moving food grown by farmers on one continent through a chain of handlers to consumers living on another continent. Information about that system is asymmetrically held, meaning that individual players—farmers, processors, distributors—may know what's going on with their part of the product or service (how it's grown, what it costs to grow it, who grew it), but nobody else does, especially the consumer. Communication is weak and trust is low, which are the major reasons why food safety advocates and sympathetic policy makers are continually clamoring for more regulation of the food system.

Imagine the members of a community-supported agriculture farm who go to their farm once a week for produce. They know the farmer and the farm, and they have complete confidence in the operation. This is the local food system at its purest and most intimate. Conversely, imagine a well-informed and well-educated shopper in a large supermarket. To gain the same level of confidence that the local farm shopper has, that consumer must read every label carefully, check all the signs, ask questions of the store personnel (who usually know nothing about the products' origin or method of production), consult dozens of Web sites and, finally, be thoroughly convinced that government-mandated labels and inspections can be trusted.

Pirog's focus is on building trust and using that trust to communicate knowledge through a statewide network whose membership runs the gamut from food banks to niche pork producers. This Iowa food system network, now in the process of being organized, will offer a more intimate and personal means by which to share knowledge from one person to the next. At its simplest level, the network brings people together on a regular basis to make face-to-face contact. This approach grows partially out of Pirog's frustration with our overreliance on technology and the Internet as a means to convey knowledge. Too many "how-to" manuals on the Web, too many experts thinking that all you have to do is view their DVD and your problems are solved, too many grants going to too many organizations that are developing volumes of training materials. "I believe in technology," Pirog said, "but I'm not going to bare my soul on some wiki!"

Tacit knowledge, unlike more formal knowledge that needs to be thought about to be shared, requires interaction and is always re-created in the present moment. If I can sit next to you and share my experience of raising free-range hogs and then tell you about a successful marketing outlet for my animals, chances are pretty good you are going to learn a lot more and be more motivated to try these methods than if you studied a dozen pamphlets distributed by your county extension office. Within a network of people who exchange information in this manner it is easier to develop and work for a shared vision of a sustainable food system.

The value of this network theory was tested very early when a small Iowa pork processor's facility burned to the ground. Within four days, the other members of the network had the plan and resources in place to rebuild the facility. That kind of response takes you far beyond the old-fashioned barn-raising model; it in fact utilizes much more sophisticated knowledge across greater distances to resolve more complex problems more rapidly.

If medieval mythology can be of use in illustrating Pirog's model, he prefers the legend of King Arthur's Roundtable. "Before King Arthur, England was nothing more than a bunch of lords and knights controlling their individual fiefdoms, none of which could get along with any other fiefdom. Though they all shared the same island, they couldn't even agree on rules for the annual inter-fiefdom joust." King Arthur, who knew as much about human nature as he did about furniture design, constructed a round table—seated there, everybody was equal and everybody was respected, regardless of his history, his lineage, or the size of his broadsword. For a good long while, at least so the legend goes, Camelot was a stellar model of a progressive civilization. Perhaps Iowa will become the same.

As high as Brahm Ahmadi's hopes are for West Oakland, he's also a realist. While he optimistically sees the community as a glass half full, he's quick to point to the half that remains empty. "There aren't a lot of technically qualified people in this community, which is why we need to invest in training," Ahmadi said, referring to the kind of skill sets he deems necessary for the new urban food economy—farmers, food store managers, and developers. Honestly appraising the current state of his constituencies' job-readiness, he ticked off a litany of health problems, family violence, lack of work experience, and poor communication skills as ongoing barriers to recruiting and retaining a competent workforce. However, he is very proud of his most recent addition. "We just hired an African American person from Memphis to be our farm manager. While he may not have as much farming background as the white job applicants we saw, he'll bring more social capital and credibility to the community. We prefer to invest in people even if it means that our production figures won't be as good as they could be."

It's this emphasis on process, on walking the talk, and on building a community team that matters most, and in Ahmadi's estimation will pay off for People's Grocery and West Oakland in the long run. The organization's philanthropic supporters don't always appreciate the primacy of process over measurable outputs, but Ahmadi reports the "social return" to his funders as well as the pounds of food, and makes a further commitment to educate them about the higher value inherent in that less quantifiable return.

Central tenets of the People's Grocery's vision are empowering the community to believe in itself and take action, and using food as a vehicle for economic control. When asked why food and not, say, housing or the environment, Ahmadi, who was originally an environmental justice organizer without a background in food, sees food as a more intimate and accessible topic. "Everyone wants to talk about it. Everyone has something to say or some experience to share. Try talking about carbon emissions or particulate matter. They are boring. People's eyes glaze over quickly. Food was a way to create businesses, jobs and, frankly, to leverage ourselves into people's lives."

That People's Grocery's staff and leaders must mirror the race and ethnicity of its constituents is an inviolate principle for Ahmadi, who is thirty-four and of Iranian descent. That is how they build trust with the West Oakland community while also educating the larger community of volunteers, funders, and liberal ally organizations. He finds himself peeved at times with "white liberal organizations that dispense charitable services but in no way reflect the people whom they are serving." Likewise, he gets upset with philanthropic organizations that do not hold their grant recipients accountable in any meaningful way for having boards of directors and staff that are nearly all white. But he makes it equally clear that people of color and their organizations will not succeed by embracing some kind of nationalistic, Black Panther–style agenda that excludes white people and allied institutions. Alternately, Ahmadi sees the large numbers of white college-age and early-twentysome-things who are dying to volunteer at People's Grocery as both a blessing and curse. "I've seen a white kid who probably grew up in New England just oozing awkwardness with people here in West Oakland. I've also had complaints from community residents when they buy produce from a white college-educated kid tending one of our farm stands. So I say to myself, 'Oh, my God, I got do something about this!'" So rather than turn these well-intentioned young folk and their youthful energy away, he has instituted antiracism training that focuses on the issues of white power and privilege, and effectively enables young people to increase their cultural competency in communities of color.

What is clear is that Ahmadi is not about division. On the contrary, he is about black and white unity, a multicultural movement for food justice, and the democratic control of the food system. After all, as he pointed out, "Obesity is a threat that transcends race and income; it's not endemic to only low-income communities of color. The environment for everyone is at risk." In the same way that Rich Pirog has created space for a diversity of food system stakeholders to communicate, establish trust, take control of their food system, and create community wealth from the ground up, Brahm Ahmadi is building the capacity of his socially and economically challenged community to control its own economic destiny through food.

CONCLUSION
FINDING THE FIRE WITHIN

Society everywhere is in conspiracy against the manhood of every one of its members. Society is a joint-stock company, in which the members agree, for the better securing of his bread to each shareholder, to surrender the liberty and culture of the eater. The virtue in most request is conformity. Self-reliance is its aversion.

—RALPH WALDO EMERSON

When confronting the ravages of the industrial food system and its quickening ability to dull our minds and our appreciation of good food, I can think of no better person to turn to than Ralph Waldo Emerson for a swift kick to our collective rear ends. Though he opposed the evils of his time—the displacement of entire Native American nations, slavery, and the forced annexation of Mexican territory—the specter of American corporatism and the manipulative hand of consumerism were still inchoate in the nineteenth-century minds of our early industrial elite. Yet Emerson sensed full well that the threat to the individual spirit sprang from many sectors, not just commercial institutions, and included dogma of any stripe, whether it was business, religion, or politics. In other words, the pressure to conform to the prevailing realities was as much the single greatest challenge to human development then as it is now.

The nineteenth-century form of individualism expressed by our foremost sage has never left the American soul. We turn to Emerson when we are suffocated by the smothering blanket of materialism and mass-minded culture that seeks to rob each of us of our essence. He has been used (and misused) at critical epochs in our nation's history to justify, among other American adventures, westward expansion, hard-driving capitalism and entrepreneurism, recent presidential campaigns, and the 1960s counterculture. But most importantly, Emerson warned us, "The centuries are conspirators against the sanity and authority of the soul," and we must "affront and reprimand the smooth mediocrity and squalid contentment of the times." He attacked complacency wherever he saw it, scolding even the college students of his era for succumbing to "a paralysis of the active faculties, which falls on young men in this country, as soon as they have finished college." His criticism could apply as well to today's college students, who grow timorous at the thought of testing their sinews in the rough-and-tumble of the world's streets and opt too soon for the sanctuary of graduate school, nervous that sixteen-plus years of schooling have left them ill-prepared for any worthy endeavor.

Our world in the 2010s is little different from the one Emerson described in the 1840s when he wrote: "We are parlor soldiers. We shun the rugged battle of fate, where strength is born." Instead of struggling against our conditions—whether imposed by poverty, privilege, or culture—we allow them to dictate the terms of our surrender. We don't do as Jean-Paul Sartre said of the imprisoned members of the French Resistance: "It is not what they do to you, it is what you do with what they do to you that matters." We may not be able to control the fate that is handed to us, but we damn sure can control our reaction to it.

Emerson's aging and ailing aunt Mary once asked ironically if there was any hope that her malady could end in death. Can we reasonably ask the same question of the industrial food system? Will it simply implode, either through some cataclysmic event or slowly, over decades, as it gradually exhausts the earth's natural resources and depletes our souls? If the industry carries on unabated and unchallenged, that may be the way our world ends, "not with a bang but with a whimper." But it will no doubt take us down with it. The poor will go first, as they always have, with no time or means to find alternatives. Those in the middle will endure a few moments longer, struggling against the certainty of their own defeat, trying not "to go gentle into that good night." And the rich, the privileged, those perched on high ground and sandbagged against the deluge, will hold out mightily to the bitter end. With their private security forces and the most advanced environmental technology capable of converting toxins to clean air and water, they will be the ones to witness the last dawn, the final sunset. But even they will find that Nature will turn the lights out on them.

So what is the antidote? Because, as my high school wrestling coach used to tell his less-than-stellar athletes, for every move there is an equally effective countermove, I can find reason to be optimistic about the contest, but only if the millions who now embrace an alternative food system can become the billions—before it's too late. To do that we must find a countermove that undercuts a system that demands our conformity, a system that clearly "is in conspiracy against the manhood [and womanhood] of every one of its members." Too many accept our food system not only as the norm but as our destiny. It's often an indifferent acceptance, but acceptance nevertheless. "Our food system works well enough," "There's plenty of food," "It tastes good," "There's no problem that I can see" are the lukewarm endorsements of the status quo. The "billions" are susceptible to a contagious cold of fast food, an epidemic of cheap and convenient meals, and a serious infection of alienation from nature. In such a state of passivity one has little inclination to engage in "the rugged battle of fate."

The argument we must make is for action, not contemplation; we must engage the food system, not presume that all is well because the food system feeds us. Hands in the soil, vegetables on the cutting board, and voices in the city council chambers will be the way that we strengthen our muscles. It will be through experience and participation, those rough but nimble teachers, that we re-create the skills we once had and now need again to attract the billions and send the Grand Inquisitor packing. "Intellectual tasting of life will not supersede muscular activity," admonished Emerson. "If a man should consider the nicety of the passage of a piece of bread down his throat, he would starve."

No doubt we find value in preparing ourselves with good teachers, whether they be our mothers or paid consultants, or in the cloistered shell of the university with its leisurely pursuit of knowledge. Learn from them, revel in those places, but turn quickly from them. Hit the road as soon as you can, armed with the knowledge paid for by your tuition, but trusting soon in your intuition. The self-sufficient man or woman is what we must become, whether born with a silver spoon in our mouth, or suckling at our mother's breast in a soup kitchen line. Thus empowered, we are then ready to join a community, make a contribution, and build the new food system.

It was a privilege to meet Maurice Small, who grew up in Cleveland's housing projects, and Dorothy Morrison, who still lives in the housing projects of Austin. Neither one has succumbed to what could have been his or her fate. Tired of seeing the same vacant lots in his city as an adult that he saw as a child, Maurice set out to put his hands in the soil in the same way that his father did. He became comfortable with his own nonconforming brand of rugged urban individualism and transferred that confidence to others. Gardens grew, but more importantly, so did the community's self-esteem. Taking an even stonier path to self-reliance, Dorothy knew hunger as a child, succumbed early to single motherhood and five children, but refused to stew in her poverty or accept the cards her fate had dealt her. Through community service and ultimately mastering her food skills and learning to improve her family's health, she began to take charge of her life and play an even greater role in helping her peers. Like Maurice, she found an inner strength from a quiet spiritual voice inside her. We don't know precisely how that dialogue went, but we do know that they both have evolved a soul as firm as a New England stone wall built from experience, faith, and confidence.

Choi Chan-Sick, the peasant rice farmer I met on the road in South Korea, verbally attacked me because I was a convenient symbol of an American policy that was attempting to impose a final solution on his country's traditional (and sacred) form of agriculture. He, like hundreds of thousands of South Korean agriculturalists and their sympathizers, was not shy in expressing his refusal to accept the fate prescribed by the global food system. To what extent he and the others win or lose will be determined over time, but you can be assured that their resistance will produce a different destiny than the one they would have submitted to if they had remained silent and polite.

Quieter and more meditative than the South Korean protestors, Bryan Vigil stands with tens of thousands of other Native Americans who have pursued, and in many cases rediscovered, the power of their own traditions as the best cure for the deleterious side effects of the white man's medicine. Casting off the sense of doom that a white person often senses on reservations (expressed by some Native Americans as the "end-time"), Bryan and his brothers and sisters are shaping something new out of the past with the hope of achieving a stable and healthy form of self-reliance. It is not likely to be a total return to a native diet—bison and native plants, for instance—but even a symbolic reconnection to the foods that sustained their ancestors for hundreds of years recenters the locus of control where it should be—in their own hands.

Robin Chesmer, Connecticut dairy farmer and entrepreneur, will not allow the corporate milk conglomerates to determine his fate any more than Lynn Walters, Santa Fe food educator, will allow another generation of children to fall prey to America's junk food culture. Both stand firm in their belief that the road to food independence and an understanding of farming can be traveled only by those willing to engage in the direct experience of both. To break down the walls between the producer and consumer will not only sell more local milk, it will bring people closer to their food, the land, and nature. The taste of real food and the sight and sound of farming will win out over the mere idea of them any day of the week. Just as there is nothing like a live "moo" delivered by a 1,200-pound Holstein from ten feet away to remind you of the sanctity of life; there is nothing like a delicious meal made from farmers' market ingredients prepared by a fourth grader to cement his or her bond with cooking. The senses lead. The ears fill with the thrum of life. The eyes confirm our subjective experience of the world around us. The nose advises the palate of what's to come, and the palate never lies. By bringing what's outside of our bodies into them, we experience a kind of ecstasy, a joy in life that, in turn, takes us outside of our bodies. We are displaced but happily so. As Emerson said, "[T]he power and genius of nature is ecstatic."

Brahm Ahmadi, Cindy Torres, and Richard Pirog are among the kind of "men and women who will renovate life and our social state." They actually believe in democracy and allow the voice of the people to thrive, even when that's inefficient and messy. Not only do they accept democracy as a first principle, they actively promote it by building the systems that will allow it to flourish. Richard is organizing the networks that facilitate effective communication between Iowa's food system stakeholders, particularly the ones who want an alternative to the corn and soybean monopoly that has ruled the land for too long. His scheme makes trust a primary ingredient in fostering connections between people that will in turn yield new ideas, innovative food and farm businesses, and an implicit faith in the place where food is produced. Similarly, Cindy and her fellow Boulder citizens have developed a county food policy council that is committed to putting forward a positive vision based on justice and sustainability for their region. Every voice counts and everyone, no matter on what side of an issue he or she may be, has the right to be heard. Though the citizens of Boulder did not go looking for a fight with the industrial food system, neither did they shun the battle. Brahm has made it clear that not only will the voices of his hardscrabble West Oakland community be heard, but community members will also own a share of their destiny. In communities of color where white-led organizations have dominated the social service sector, he has argued persuasively that those who are victims of oppression and racism must be allowed, and must allow themselves, to take charge of their future.

As if anticipating the creation of Dostoevsky's Grand Inquisitor, Emerson wrote, "The one serious and formidable thing in nature is a will. Society is servile from want of will, and therefore the world wants saviors and religions." The people whose lives run through these pages are blessed with ample will. They do not need religion or similar institutions to fall down before, but draw instead on their faith and values to find the strength they need to help themselves and others. They may be, as their numbers grow, the leaders who make the millions billions. Let us see. Let us hope.

The columnist Ellen Goodman once wrote that she did not regard the nearly infinite choice of food items in today's supermarkets as an emblem of her freedom as a consumer, but rather as a chain around her neck that enslaved her to a never-ending onslaught of largely superfluous food items that left her confused and disoriented, rambling about the supermarket, finding nothing to eat. A large supermarket has tens of thousands of different food items to choose from, and the food industry introduces as many as 15,000 new food items every year. Holding aside the health and dietary consequences of our food choices, which of course are enormous, how are we to choose from this maddening array of food? Has this so-called abundance made our lives simpler, or simply crazy?

On a personal level, I decided to narrow my range of options, and in so doing, take a more mindful approach to what I eat. I am trying to eat locally and seasonally—and, as much as possible, assemble my daily menus from an admittedly narrower—but, happily, tastier—range of choices that are closer at hand. I start with our garden and then move to the farmers' market for the produce we eat. We buy beef from a New Mexico rancher whom we know personally and whose cows are raised entirely on grass. As discussed earlier, I've been to the facility where the cows are slaughtered; it's locally owned, employs ten people in a small town where every job counts, operates humanely and, on a good day, is able to slaughter only four cows compared to the thousands that are slaughtered daily in a large corporate meatpacking plant.

Not all our food is local. I buy Organic Valley milk at the supermarket, which is produced by dairies in Colorado as well as ones all across the country. I've investigated that farmer-owned co-op and I'm convinced that it protects the environment, the cows, and the safety of its milk more than the factory dairy farms that operate in New Mexico. A trip to Whole Foods is a treat that we can afford to indulge in only every other month. We buy coffee from a fair trade company out of Massachusetts. I know its founders and trust the business. The rest of the time we're shopping at Albertson's, the national chain supermarket, for such things as bananas, cereal and, of course, beer and wine, favoring the small regional breweries and vintners, though I must admit that the product of the latter takes a bit of getting used to.

The simplifying act is to start with what we have first and to put together simple meals around those foods. A whole, free-range chicken from Whole Foods was the accessory to the carrots, parsnips, and onions from our garden. New Mexico beef will anchor the green chiles, tomatoes, and potatoes from the garden for tomorrow night's stew. We store produce, can produce, freeze produce, and (when the food dryer is working) dry produce. Like little squirrels storing nuts, we stash food everywhere.

I'm not trying to imitate Barbara Kingsolver or eat only the 100-mile diet. I'm not a food purist, nor do I while away my days in a state of hyperanxiety over the safety, origin, or method of production of all the food I buy. I love to garden; it's my recreation, my fitness club, my calisthenics. It's also the focal point for as many meals as possible. I like farmers and ranchers. I spend time getting to know them, and sometimes, much to their chagrin, even write about them. I learn about other foods—what's good and what's not—when I have time. I don't read labels obsessively, but if I can't pronounce most of the words in the ingredients list, I generally put it back on the shelf. When I haven't been fortunate enough to have my own garden, I've joined a community garden, shopped more at the farmers' market, and bought a share in a CSA.

When we sit down to dinner, my wife and I often count the number of items on our plates that are "local." Many nights we hit 100 percent and will toast that fact with a glass of wine; other nights it's much less. But every night we strive for at least a token morsel of something local, even if it's a dried-up clove of garlic from last year's garden. This is the emblem of our freedom and the way we celebrate life's simple pleasures.

But there's one more facet to the process of simplification, and it's not so simple. In my opinion, it's not enough to satisfy your own desire for simplicity and good food, and to only be an informed food *consumer*. You need to be an informed food *citizen* as well. This means two things. The first is that if you believe that you should have the best and healthiest food available, then shouldn't everybody, regardless of income? This is what we call "food justice." I think it is worthwhile to align your charitable giving and actions with your values and personal practices, and to that end I believe that we need to think a little more deeply about who and what we support if we are going to achieve food justice. Rather than writing another check to the local food bank—which, while worthy, addresses only the immediate need and not the failure of the underlying system that perpetuates that need—it may be worth looking at programs that support beginning, socially disadvantaged farmers, or initiatives that try to protect the area's precious farmland, or projects that help people acquire the skills and confidence they need to become self-reliant. Perhaps you can take more direct action by pulling together a group of people from your school, neighborhood, or faith community to buy shares for low-income families at an area CSA, or otherwise encouraging the purchase of local bounty by all.

The second characteristic of good food citizenship has to do with public policy. At city halls and in our state legislatures, food and farm advocacy organizations and our elected officials are doing more to hold the industrial food system accountable for its actions and place it under a regulatory yoke that will prevent further harm. In spite of the conservative propensity to downsize the public sector, the only thing that will rein in Big Food is Big Government. Similarly, public policy is being used to promote the development of the alternative food system. Publicly supported efforts to prioritize local and regional farming, healthier and locally grown food for students in our public schools, and more opportunities for low-income people to better feed their families must be encouraged and expanded. Private charities and local farms are only part of the solution. As good food citizens, we need to speak up for policies and practices that promote a just and sustainable food system for all.

So there you have it, my recipe for a simpler, self-reliant, and more fulfilling life. Eat local and seasonal, support causes that are promoting the same for everybody, and get loud with your lawmakers.

LIVING LIFE VIVIDLY

Emerson's rant against conformity, his affirmation of self-reliance, and my embrace of simplicity constitute slightly different roads that one might follow to cast off the manacles of the industrial food system. Emerson and I both urge society's members to reject "business as usual," while I hope for a new revival in American individualism that will ignite a dramatic expansion of the alternative food system—one based on health, justice, democracy, and sustainability.

At a very realistic level, I nevertheless worry about how any of us will find the time to take more responsibility for producing and preparing food. Sometimes by necessity, but often by choice, too many of us have permitted our lives to become severely circumscribed by the encumbrances of too much work and a consumerist set of leisure pursuits. Whether we are an upwardly mobile professional couple with our minds and bodies wired to multiple electronic gizmos, or a blue-collar family working multiple jobs to make ends meet, we trade the pursuit of the heavenly bread for the earthly bread.

This pursuit is made possible, at least in our present-day culture, by so-called advances in technology, wealth, productivity, and the availability of low-cost labor. I can become a successful law firm partner as long as there are others to care for my children, mow my lawn, build my ski chalet in the mountains, and grow and cook my food—all earning wages, of course, that are low enough not to impinge on my lifestyle. But what do I forfeit by allowing others to care for me? I must trust the system that is capable of churning out my basic necessities and, in effect, give away my control of these items to others. And as we have come to see, the forfeiture of responsibility to the industrial food system comes close to making a deal with the devil.

But I think we lose something else that is perhaps more essential when we turn over all manual labor to others, when in fact the only time we sweat is in the gym, not in the garden. What we lose is our self-reliance, our engagement with the wider world of community and nature; and foremost of all, we run the very real risk of losing our soul. Taking on Adam Smith's rationalization of production, Emerson says, "Society pays heavily for the economy it derives from the division of labor." He goes on at some length to describe his "Representative Man," who seems to embody a person of rugged individualism equipped with sufficient strength, skill, and intelligence to survive handily on the frontier. He compares individuals such as that—sometimes referring to people of French-Canadian or Native American ancestry—to others whom he labels "the emaciated broken-hearted pin or buckle or stock-maker, more helpless the further the division is carried." Speaking in less literal terms and fast-forwarding 150 years, we can safely say that the greater the distance between ourselves and the necessities of life, the greater will be the alienation of the soul, and greater yet will be the power of the industrial food system to direct the choices we make about our food, our health, and our communities.

As much as I can commit to vigorously pursuing the development of a dominant alternative food system, I must honestly acknowledge the difficulty in ever attaining that goal. Why? It may be that the Grand Inquisitor was right; humankind is weak and ultimately craves the miracle, mystery, and authority that the industrial food system so ably offers. It may be we humans cannot tolerate our freedom, nor will we ever be capable of firmly grasping morality, also known as the "heavenly bread," because the seductions of the "earthly bread"—property, money, and technology— are simply too powerful. The Grand Inquisitor offers us a realistic portrait of humankind that is the antithesis of the one suggested by both Christ and Emerson.

Being the practical man that I am at heart, I always like to have a Plan B. In other words, it may not be a bad idea to have a hedge in the event that the Grand Inquisitor was right. To that end I found some guidance from the British writer (and one time New Mexico resident) D. H. Lawrence, one of the more progressive observers of human nature that the early twentieth century produced. Lawrence was one of those critics who found in favor of the Grand Inquisitor, and he, in all likelihood, would have come down on the side of the Inquisitor's contemporary embodiment, Alston Whitlaw. In short, Lawrence concluded that Jesus Christ got it wrong. "Jesus loved mankind for what it ought to be, free and limitless," says Lawrence. "The Grand Inquisitor loves [humanity] for what it is, with all its limitations." By expecting so much of human beings—challenging them to choose the heavenly bread over the earthly bread, for instance—Christianity has made "man like a horse harnessed to a load he cannot possibly pull." We are too vicious and too selfish ever to share the bread, and must therefore "hand the common bread over to some absolute authority" such as a ruling or corporate elite. Looking back over a nearly unbroken history of monarchies, despots, demagogic politicians, and modern-day mega-corporations, it may be hard to argue with Lawrence's point. Without the control of one final and accepted authority, all would be in chaos and all would ultimately starve. Or so the argument goes.

Not long ago we saw these ideas played out on the national political stage. Following 9/11, with the Patriot Act and the abuse of civil liberties that followed, the American people submitted like never before to authority. At first we believed it was in our self-interest—America had been attacked, thousands had died, and we were scared. But then we slowly discovered that those who are granted an uncommon amount of trust in times of emergency don't easily relinquish that additional authority when the emergency has abated. The statement "We know what's best for you" is always on the lips of current or future tyrants.

Yes, this is humankind's weakness, a tendency to bow down to authority for life's basic necessities and security, and to forfeit our freedom, especially when a reasonable case for our vulnerability can be made. It is what Lawrence refers to as "the bitter limitation of the mass of men." It is for the earthly bread, the literal food that sustains life, that we may degrade ourselves. But this is where Lawrence presents another choice, another way out, if you will, that may free us emotionally and spiritually, if not literally, from the grip of the industrial food system. While we may be dependent to some degree on the earthly bread, he acknowledges, it doesn't mean that we can't also pursue the heavenly bread that promotes "[t]rue living [and] fills us with vivid life."

Lawrence finds a unity of sorts between the sacred and the secular in, of all things, the sowing of land and the harvesting of crops. "In sowing the seed man has his contact with earth, with sun and rain. . . . In the awareness of the springing of the corn he has his ever-renewed consciousness of miracle, wonder, and mystery. . . . Again, in the reaping and the harvest are another contact with earth and sun . . . and the joy of harvest-home." Like Emerson before him, like Maurice Small after him, and like millions of others for whom "contact with earth" transports them to both heavenly and earthly stations, Lawrence reminds us that life is physical, active, hard, and "the sweat of the brow is the heavenly butter."

Will the industrial food system crash from its own weight and be consumed by its own flames? It may not matter if we can learn how to live life more vividly, more physically, and with more communal unity. Seizing as much of our sustenance back from the earthly masters as we can—through locally and sustainably produced food, food we prepare from whole ingredients ourselves, supported by policies that we, the people, shape—may be as much as we can ever know of paradise on earth, and joyfully so.

NOTES

Information for this book was gathered from four basic sets of sources: on-site interviews, my own reporting based on firsthand observation of events, background reading from the texts listed below, and numerous periodicals, data sets, reports, and research publications, also cited below.

CHAPTER 1: A FOOD STORY FOR OUR TIMES

For further reading: Terry Eagleton, "Freedom by Necessity," *Lapham's Quarterly,* Winter 2010; George Lakoff, *Don't Think of an Elephant: Know Your Values and Frame the Debate* (White River Junction, VT: Chelsea Green, 2004); Robert D. Richardson Jr., *Emerson: The Mind on Fire* (Berkeley and Los Angeles: University of California Press, 1995); Wayne Roberts, *The Non-Nonsense Guide to World Food* (Toronto: New Internationalist, 2008); and Joan Dye Gussow, *Chicken Little, Tomato Sauce and Agriculture* (New York: Bootstrap, 1991).

CHAPTER 2: THE FIGHT FOR THE SOUL OF THE AMERICAN FOOD SYSTEM

Information on "Good Food" from an article in the *Rochester Democrat and Chronicle,* September 5, 2007; and from the W. K. Kellogg Foundation Web site and Food and Society Update, www.ola.wkkf.org/fasupdate/2007/march/first.htm.

USDA National Agriculture Statistics Service, 2007 Agriculture Census. www .agcensus.usda.gov/publications/2007/index.asp.

Additional information on organic food sales and production provided by the Western Region Sustainable Agriculture Research and Education agency, www .wsare.usu.edu.

Information on direct marketing is from *Facts on Direct-to-Consumer Food Marketing* (USDA Agricultural Marketing Service, May 2009).

Additional information provided by *Local and Fresh Foods,* a report of the market research firm Package Facts, as reported by the School Nutrition Association, June 2007.

Figures on farmers' markets are from the USDA; on CSAs from personal discussion with Elizabeth Henderson; on farm-to-school programs from personal discussion with Marion Kalb; on farm-to-college programs from the Real Food Challenge, www.realfoodchallenge.org.

Food import figures were reported in the *Sacramento Bee,* June 16, 2007.

"The Rise of the Locavore," *Business Week,* May 20, 2008.

Information on what constitutes "local" was reported by *USA Today,* October 27, 2008.

Information on packaging and marketing practices reported in *Advertising Age,* June 8, 2007.

Information about Dannon yogurt was contained in a press release from Health Care without Harm, February 26, 2009.

Information about Sodexo's size and employment was contained in a Sodexo press release, February 11, 2009; information on charitable projects was placed on the Comfood Listserv, April 6, 2008.

Information about Starbucks was contained in job notice issued by Starbucks and placed on the Comfood Listserv, November 2, 2008.

Information about the food price index from the *Economist,* December 8, 2007.

Salt Lake City Deseret News, April 20, 2008.

Information on the 2008 U.S. Health and Human Services Department obesity study reported in the *Philadelphia Inquirer,* May 6, 2008.

Information about Albuquerque public schools provided by the New Mexico Food and Agriculture Policy Council.

Paul Roberts, *The End of Food* (Boston: Houghton Mifflin, 2009).

Fyodor Dostoevsky, *The Brothers Karamazov,* trans. Richard Pevear and Larissa Volokhonsky (New York: Farrar, Straus and Giroux, 1990).

Fyodor Dostoevsky, *The Grand Inquisitor,* ed. Jerry S. Wasserman (Columbus, OH: Charles E. Merrill, 1970).

Sigmund Freud, cited in Wasserman's edition of Dostoevsky, *The Grand Inquisitor.*

CHAPTER 3: THE INDUSTRIAL FOOD SYSTEM

Information about EPA, agricultural chemicals, and CAFOs provided by *High Country News,* December 22, 2008.

Information on New Mexico dairy CAFOs from National Public Radio, December 9, 2009; and from reporting done by Mark Winne for essays that appeared in *Growing a Healthy Food System: Food and Agriculture in New Mexico* (Santa Fe: New Mexico Food and Agriculture Policy Council, 2005) and on AlterNet, October 29, 2008.

"Maryland Is Turning Pollution Spotlight to Its Huge Poultry Industry," *New York Times,* November 29, 2008.

Journal of the American Medical Association, as reported in Michael Pollan, "Our Decrepit Food Factories," *New York Times Magazine,* December 16, 2007.

Information on antibiotics in livestock from "Administration Seeks to Restrict Antibiotics in Livestock," *New York Times,* July 14, 2009; *Putting Meat on the*

Table: Industrial Farm Animal Production in America (Philadelphia: Pew Charitable Trusts, April 29, 2008).

Other sources consulted for livestock information are Nicholas D. Kristof, "Our Pigs, Our Food, Our Health," *New York Times*, March 12, 2009; Pollan, "Our Decrepit Food Factories"; and "The Ugly Truth Behind Organic Food," AlterNet, May 14, 2009.

Information on farm workers and agriprocessors from "Kosher Plant Is Accused of Inhumane Slaughter," *New York Times*, September 5, 2008; and "Meatpacker Is Fined Nearly $10 Million," *New York Times*, October 30, 2008.

Mars candy story as reported in "Mars Sets Goal for Sustainable Cocoa Sources," *Washington Post*, April 10, 2009.

Information on McDonald's from a press release issued by Investor Environmental Health Network, March 31, 2009.

Adoption of Genetically Engineered Crops in the U.S. (Washington, DC: Economic Research Service, USDA, July 2, 2008).

Mike Mack, op-ed, *Newsweek*, December 31, 2008.

Monsanto's profits as reported in "Monsanto Profit More than Doubles," CNNMoney.com, January 7, 2009.

Robert Paarlberg, *Starved for Science: How Biotechnology Is Being Kept out of Africa* (Cambridge, MA: Harvard College Press, 2008).

The story on David Chicoine was reported in "When Big Business and Academia Mix, Where Is the Line?" *Lincoln Journal Star*, April 25, 2009.

Information on the Bill and Melinda Gates Foundation was reported in "Gates Grant Will Help Danforth Center Fight Hunger," *St. Louis Post-Dispatch*, January 7, 2009.

Katha Pollit, "The Kindness of Strangers," *Nation*, February 23, 2009.

Information about the World Food Prize was contained in an invitation sent to Mark Winne.

Kelly Brownell and Kenneth Warner, "The Perils of Ignoring History: Big Tobacco Played Dirty and Millions Died: How Similar Is Big Food?" *Millbrook Quarterly* 87, no. 1 (2009).

John F. Brock III statement appeared in "Praise, Advice and Reminders of the Sour Economy for Graduates," *New York Times*, June 14, 2009.

Tom Keane, "Choose Local Food for the Taste? Sure. But If You're Convinced You're Saving the World, Think Again," *Boston Globe*, June 28, 2009.

Stephen J. Dubner, "Do We Really Need a Few Billion Locavores?" *New York Times*, June 9, 2008.

George F. Will, *Washington Post*, December 27, 2007.

"Meatpacker Puts Stamp on Europe," *New York Times*, May 7, 2009.

Derrick Z. Jackson, "Burger King's Greasy Campaign," *Boston Globe*, December 8, 2008.

Information on Monsanto from Donald Barlett and James Steele, "Monsanto's Harvest of Fear," *Vanity Fair*, May 2008.

GMO and Hawaii reported by Bret Yager, "GMO Bills to Reignite Debate in Legislature," *Stephens Media,* February 8, 2009.

GMO and Montana reported by Kahrin Deines, "Seed Sampling Bill Gets a Hearing in Montana," for the Associated Press, March 19, 2009.

GMO and Boulder County, Colorado, information provided by Cindy Torres through personal communication.

CHAPTER 4: MAURICE SMALL AND THE GREENING OF CLEVELAND

Information in this chapter comes from interviews with Maurice Small, Cleveland city councilman Joe Cimperman, Case Western Reserve University food service director Joe Gentile, Brad Masi at the New Agrarian Center (Oberlin College), and other community leaders in Cleveland, Ohio.

Information about Bon Appetite gathered from company press releases, Web sites, and brochures.

Ralph Waldo Emerson, "Self-Reliance," in *Ralph Waldo Emerson: Nature and Selected Essays* (New York: Penguin, 2003).

CHAPTER 5: ME AND MY MEAT

Small sections of this chapter have appeared in *In These Times, Sun Monthly,* and on AlterNet.

Information for this chapter was gathered during the course of reporting confined cattle and dairy operations in eastern New Mexico. Interviews were conducted with dozens of farmers, ranchers, community residents, and public officials. Most of them asked me to leave their names out of my story, including one farmer and long-standing member of the community who told me that he had endured several threatening remarks from the region's agribusiness representatives for talking to me.

"A Bumper Crop," *Washington Post,* June 17, 2007.

Information about Oklahoma and hog CAFOs was provided by the Kerr Center and through personal communication with one of its staff members, Anita Poole.

Information about the distance traveled by locally produced and directly marketed cattle/beef compared to that which goes through the industrial and regional system was provided by Farm to Table, a Santa Fe–based nonprofit food organization.

Union of Concerned Scientists, *Greener Pastures—How Grass-Fed Beef and Milk Contribute to Healthy Eating,* March 7, 2006, www.ucsusa.org/assets/documents/food_and_agriculture/greener-pastures.

CHAPTER 6: THE FARMER'S COW

A few paragraphs of this chapter originally appeared in "Enterprise Working to Keep Local Dairy Farms Viable," *Hartford Courant,* July 5, 2009.

Information for this chapter was gathered from on-site interviews with Robin Chesmer and other Connecticut dairy farmers.

Information about farmland preservation in Connecticut was gathered from the Connecticut Department of Agriculture, the Working Lands Alliance, and the Natural Resources Conservation Service (USDA).

Hartford Courant, February 4, 2009.

CHAPTER 7: GOD DIDN'T MAKE NACHOS

All the information for this chapter was gathered during the course of interviews with staff and participants of the Sustainable Food Center and that organization's Happy Kitchen Program in Austin, Texas.

CHAPTER 8: HEALTHY SCHOOLS GROW HEALTHY KIDS

All the information for this chapter was gathered from interviews in Santa Fe, New Mexico.

CHAPTER 9: GETTING OUR HEADS ABOVE THE PLATE

All the information for this chapter was gathered during the course of a visit to Bates College in Lewiston, Maine, and from the Bates College and Bates Contemplates Food Initiative Web site.

CHAPTER 10: FOOD SOVEREIGNTY

Portions of the South Korea section of this chapter previously appeared on the *Nation* online.

Information about the Myskoke Nation in Oklahoma comes from an interview with Vicky Karhu, who is a member of that community.

Information about Hawaii comes from interviews with Hawaiian community leaders and food activists conducted during a visit to O'ahu and Kauai.

Information about the Jicarilla Apache was gathered during the course of reporting on that nation's food initiatives for the New Mexico Food and Agriculture Policy Council.

Information for the section on South Korea was gathered from a 2007 visit to that country, and from interviews conducted during that time; rice production and subsidy figures are from the USDA.

Updates on the current state of the South Korean/U.S. FTA come from an August 23, 2009, entry at Wikipedia.org.

CHAPTER 11: FOOD CITIZENS, UNITE!

Portions of this chapter have appeared in *YES! Magazine* (Spring 2009).

Information about New Mexico; Boulder, Colorado; Cleveland; and Connecticut was gathered on-site in the course of reporting or conducting training sessions in those places. Interviews for Missoula, Montana, and Portland, Oregon, were conducted via phone. All interviews were conducted on-site or by phone with the people identified in this chapter.

Additional information about Boulder, Colorado, was provided by Cindy

Torres, including memos, postings on Huffington Post, and material from the *Boulder Daily Camera.*

CHAPTER 12: REFLECTIONS ON FOOD DEMOCRACY
All information for this chapter was gathered from face-to-face interviews with Richard Pirog and Brahm Ahmadi.

CONCLUSION: FINDING THE FIRE WITHIN
Emerson, *Nature and Selected Essays.*
Emerson, *Emerson's Complete Essays* (New York: Carlton House, n.d.).
D. H. Lawrence, *Selected Literary Criticism* (New York: Viking, 1970).